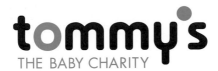
tommy's
THE BABY CHARITY

Tommy's guide to pre-pregnancy care

**A complete handbook to help you plan
your pregnancy and give your baby
the best possible start in life**

By Penny Tassoni

Author	Penny Tassoni
Editor	Mary James
Project Manager	Charlotte Davies

Designed by AMR Ltd, Basingstoke
Printed by Wyndeham Keyne Print, Milton Keynes, UK

Photograph credits:
Brocklebank-Scott, Diana: page 53
Bubbles: pages 9, 10, 11, 15 (x2), 17, 18, 19 (lower), 20, 21 (x2), 23 (x3), 24, 25, 26, 31, 32 (x2), 33, 34, 36 (x4), 42, 44 (x2), 46, 54–55, 58, 59, 60, 65, 68, 69 (x2), 72, 76 (right), 80, 87 (x2)
Citizens Advice Bureau: page 90
Greg Evans: pages 7, 28, 41, 48, 76 (left)
Powerstock: pages 42, 50
Rex Features: page 13
John Ridley: page 19 (upper)

Artwork credits:
Josephine Blake: for pages 15, 47, 50, 59, 60 (x3)
David Woodroffe: for pages 11, 13, 14, 16, 17, 28, 39, 72, 73, 83

Published in 2003 by Tommy's, the baby charity
Nicholas House
3 Laurence Pountney Hill
London
EC4R 0BB

British Library Catologuing in Publication Data
A catalogue record for this book is available from the British Library.

ISBN 0-9546426-0-0

Disclaimer
The author and Tommy's have ensured that this book was checked by experts in the field and to the best of their knowledge was considered to be accurate at the time of printing.

Contents

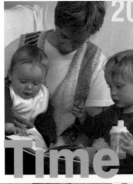

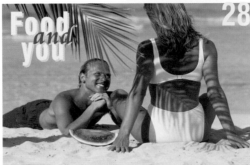

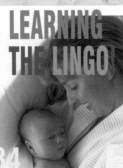

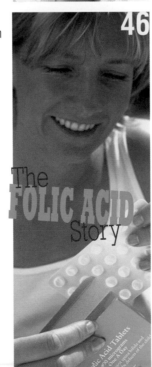

3

Contents

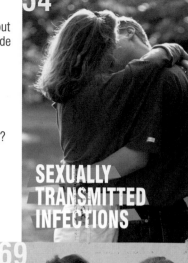

SEXUALLY
TRANSMITTED
INFECTIONS

54

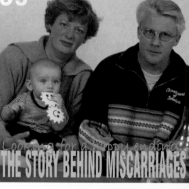

THE STORY BEHIND MISCARRIAGES

69

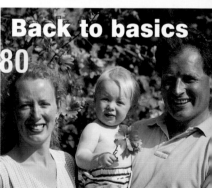

Back to basics

80

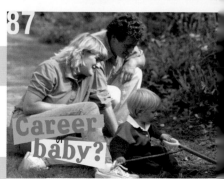

Career or baby?

87

Foreword

Beginning or adding to a family is an adventure. There is much information available about being pregnant, but many people feel there is not much for those who are thinking about getting going. This book is designed to get you off to a flying start by providing you with up-to-date information about conception which will help you to be in the best possible shape for having a baby.

If you are thinking about starting a family, or just want to know a little bit more, then this book is for you. It is packed with articles, tips and advice from some top experts. You will also hear from others who have taken the journey already. The aim is to allow you to browse through the book and take in as much information as you feel you need, without taking away the fun of it all.

We hope that you will enjoy the journey that may lead you into parenthood. Good luck!

Mr Ian Fergusson FRCS FRCOG
Founder and Trustee, Tommy's, the baby charity

Tommy's thank you

Tommy's would like to thank Team Toxo for their wonderful fundraising efforts in the London Marathon 2002. The money raised by this team is dedicated to increasing the awareness and prevention of Toxoplasmosis and has been used to promote and market this book as part of that campaign. A special mention goes to Diana Brocklebank Scott and Anthony Scott without whom Team Toxo would not have been formed and whose support and encouragement have been invaluable to all involved in this project.

Perhaps you could consider helping Tommy's. We are committed to providing our information and education programme free of charge, as we aim to give every pregnancy the best possible chance of a healthy outcome. To help us continue to provide information at no charge to parents-to-be, including books like these, **please consider making a contribution to our programme**. Every gift, no matter how small, will help us to produce more books and information products like this one, and help us save babies' lives.

Phone our donation line on 0870 777 76 76, or fill out the form overleaf.

Help save babies' lives

Tommy's exists to save babies' lives. We fund pioneering research into miscarriage, stillbirth and premature birth and provide information on pregnancy health.

Our information and education programme is free of charge, so we are able to provide everyone with the best possible chance of having a healthy pregnancy and a healthy baby. But we need your help.

☐ **I'd like to help Tommy's give every baby the chance to be born healthy**

Name	Address
	Postcode
Telephone	Email

☐ **I'd like to give regularly to Tommy's from my bank account**

Bank name	Bank Address
	Postcode
Name of account holder	

Sort code ☐☐ ☐☐ ☐☐   Bank a/c no ☐☐☐☐☐☐☐☐

Please pay Tommy's, the baby charity, the sum of £ [_____] per month/year (delete as appropriate)

starting from 0 1 / M M / Y Y and until further notice (Please ensure the start date is at least one month from today's date)

For bank use only, please quote reference

To the National Westminster bank plc, PO Box 7929, 91 Westminster Bridge Road, London SE1 7ZB for the credit of Tommy's, the baby charity account no. 26142058, sort code 60-60-04

☐ **I'd like to make a single gift**

I enclose a cheque/postal order/CAF voucher payable to Tommy's, the baby charity ☐

Please debit my Visa/Mastercard/Switch/CAF card ☐

☐☐☐☐ ☐☐☐☐ ☐☐☐☐ ☐☐☐☐

Start date M M / Y Y   Expiry date M M / Y Y   Issue no (Switch only) ☐☐

giftaid it   ☐ I'd like my gift to be worth 28% more to Tommy's at no extra cost to me!

Tommy's can claim back the tax on your gift, increasing its value at no extra cost to you. You need to be a UK taxpayer, paying as much tax as we'd be claiming. If you're not a UK taxpayer, or don't currently pay enough tax, please tick here ☐

Signature	Date

We will not pass your details to other organisations or charities.
☐ *Please tick this box if you do not wish to receive further mailings from Tommy's.*

**Please return this form to
Tommy's, the baby charity,
FREEPOST LON1053, London EC4B 4BR.**

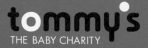

6

TOMMY'S THE BABY CHARITY is a registered charity no 1060508

PCB/04

Contraception

SO YOU'RE THINKING ABOUT GETTING PREGNANT? FINE, BUT WHAT ABOUT STOPPING CONTRACEPTION AND HOW EASY IT IS TO GET PREGNANT? WE ANSWER YOUR QUESTIONS.

For many women, starting to think about babies is both scary and exciting. You may know that you want to try for a baby in the next few months or you may be hoping to wait a little longer. But planning ahead is definitely worthwhile.

Thinking about contraception is a good starting point. Maria Simpson, an expert reproduction and sexual health nurse explains, ' Women who are taking the pill or who are having contraceptive injections need to allow enough time for their body to return back to being fertile. This means that if you are due for a repeat prescription or injection, it may be as well to talk it through with the doctor or family planning advisor who can then suggest alternative means of contraception such as condoms.'

LEARNING ABOUT YOUR BODY CLOCK

As well as looking at stopping contraception, Maria also suggests that women use this time to learn about their bodies and that they start to take folic acid. 'It is a good idea for all women to get to know their body clocks as this can help them work out when they are most fertile.' She goes onto add, 'One of the most common myths is that ovulation takes place 14 days after the first day of your last period, but this will not necessarily be the case for all women as it very much depends on your cycle length.'

IRREGULAR PERIODS

While some women's bodies work like clocks, this is not the case for everyone. Many women find that after stopping the pill or injections, their periods are irregular at first, which can come as a surprise. Maria suggests that noting other changes to the body might be helpful. 'Cervical fluid becomes much thinner and clearer just before ovulation, almost like egg white'.

It is also possible to find out when you are about to ovulate by learning about your body's temperature changes. If you want to chart your temperature, take your temperature before getting out of bed in the morning. The temperature of your body drops slightly immediately before ovulation, but rises to a higher level when ovulation has taken place.

For more information on conception, see page 16. If you are planning to get pregnant then start taking folic acid.

A QUICK GUIDE TO STOPPING CONTRACEPTION

Once they have decided to start a family, many couples are anxious to know how quickly they can stop contraception and get on with it! Our quick guide gives you a summary of information, although you may also want to visit your family planning clinic or doctor to find out exactly what's best for you.

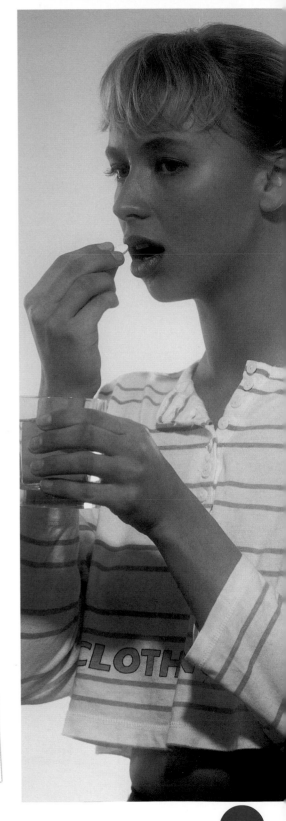

Fertility facts

85% of couples conceive within one year

50% of couples manage it in two to three months

10 to 15% of couples seek medical advice for conception

Method	What do I need to do?
The Pill (Combined Oral Contraceptive)	➤ Finish the packet you are on. ➤ Many doctors advise that you should delay trying to conceive for two to three months so that your body is back to its pattern. Fertility levels normally return during this time. ➤ Use alternative forms of contraception such as condoms. ➤ Most women are pregnant after stopping the pill within a year.
Progesterone Pill	➤ Finish the packet you are on. ➤ Many doctors advise that you should wait for one period before trying to conceive. ➤ Fertility levels return quickly.
Depo-Provera (Injectable hormones)	➤ Do not renew your injections. ➤ It will take up to twelve weeks for the effects of the injections to wear off. Many women also find that it can take as long as a year before they conceive. ➤ Seek advice from your doctor or family planning clinic.
Progesterone implants e.g. Norplant	➤ This is usually long-term contraception, but can be reversed. ➤ Make an appointment with your doctor to have the implants removed. This is usually a quick procedure done with a local anaesthetic. Fertility levels return quite quickly with 40% of women conceiving with four months. ➤ You might be advised to wait for a period before trying to conceive.
Coil (Intrauterine Device, IUD)	➤ Make an appointment with your doctor or family planning clinic to have it removed. ➤ You might be advised to wait until your next period before starting to conceive. Fertility levels should not be affected.
Condoms (male and female)	➤ Stop using them when you are ready to try for a baby. These don't affect your fertility levels.
Diaphragm and Cap	➤ Stop using them when you are ready to try for a baby. These don't affect your fertility levels.
Rhythm/temperature method	➤ This method does not affect your fertility levels. Aim now to have sex during the times when you were previously abstaining.
Withdrawal	➤ This method does not affect your fertility levels. While in theory, you could have become pregnant using withdrawal method alone, increase your chances now by not withdrawing.
Spermicide	➤ This method does not affect your fertility levels. Stop using spermicide, although consider in future that this method alone may not prevent an unwanted pregnancy.

DR JANE TODD ANSWERS YOUR QUESTIONS

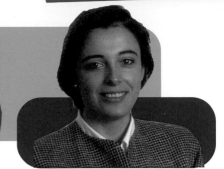

We have been trying for a baby for eleven months now and I am beginning to panic. How long should I leave it before getting help?

First of all don't panic. Not only will stress reduce your chances of conceiving, you should also know that many couples take twelve months or so. You may, however, wish to consult your doctor, if only for some reassurance, if you have not conceived after twelve months. Don't be embarrassed about going. It is thought that between 10 and 15% of couples talk to their doctors about their concerns about fertility.

My new partner wants us to start a family, but he has had a vasectomy. Is there any way in which we can start a family?

About a third of vasectomies are reversed successfully and so your partner may wish to discuss this option with his doctor. If reversal fails, you both might then consider other options, such as using donor sperm. Your doctor should be able to advise you.

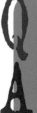

I am 35 years old and we are thinking about starting a family. I am a little unsure about how long we can wait, although I know that many women are having babies into their forties.

First, there is no perfect age to have a baby, as beside the physical aspect, you will also be making an emotional and even a financial commitment. In terms of fertility, there are many factors that affect women's ability to conceive including diet and lifestyle. Age is another. Older women usually take longer to conceive and miscarriage rates can be higher. Whilst a woman in her mid twenties may conceive in two to three months, a woman in her late thirties may need a year or more. This does not mean that you will not be able to have a baby when you are in your forties, but many experts now advise women to start earlier rather than later. So if you feel otherwise ready, you may wish to go for it now!

I think I'm pregnant. Shall I keep on taking the pill?

First of all get a pregnancy test done. If positive, you should stop taking the pill immediately. But don't worry unnecessarily. There is at present no evidence that exposure to the hormones will harm the baby, although you might still like to talk to your doctor.

I came off the pill and fell pregnant before having a 'real' period. Is the baby in any danger?

Ideally it's a good idea to let the body settle down to a normal pattern and to allow the man-made hormones that are in the pill to have worked their way out of your system. Having periods again also means that it is easier to monitor the pregnancy accurately as there may be some question as to how advanced the baby's development is. Fortunately, there is no current evidence to suggest that the baby will have been harmed in any way.

I have been on the pill for several years. Will this mean that it will take longer for my body to get back to having normal periods?

There is no evidence to suggest that being on the pill for a long time makes any difference. Some women's periods get back to a regular pattern after two or three months, while for others it can take a little longer. Do, however, see your doctor if you have not had a period after 3 months.

FACT OR FICTION?

There are many myths about getting pregnant. Test your knowledge in our quick quiz:

1 You have to have an orgasm to conceive
True or False

2 You can't get pregnant if you are breastfeeding
True or False

3 It's not possible to get pregnant the first time you have sex
True or False

4 Sperm can survive for up to seven days
True or False

5 You can't get pregnant if your partner has not penetrated you
True or False

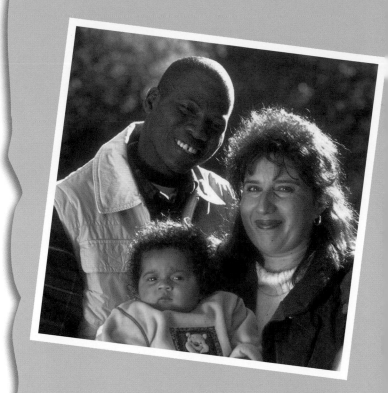

Sadie, 34, and Harvey, 36, now have Michael who is nine months old.

'I had been on the pill on and off since I was eighteen. After we decided to start a family, I was very excited and stopped taking the pill as soon as I'd finished the packet I was on. It took a while for my periods to settle down and so although we had hoped that it would happen quickly, it didn't quite go like that. After six months, I remember feeling a bit worried that I hadn't fallen pregnant, especially as several of my friends got pregnant.

It started to get a bit stressful and although I tried not to think too much about it, there was a point where every time I stepped outside the front door I seemed to notice a pram or pushchair.

In the end, it was while we were on holiday that I realised I was pregnant. It took us nine months, which I now know is really normal, although at the time it felt that it might never happen. Looking back, I wish that I had plucked up the courage to talk to the doctor about coming off the pill. That way I might have found out more about how long it takes most couples to conceive. I think that would have taken a lot of stress out of it for us and also helped us with other advice, like eating healthily and taking folic acid. We're hoping to try for another baby soon, but this time I have already been up to the family planning clinic for advice.'

ANSWERS

1 False. It might be nice, but it's not a requirement!

2 False. While breastfeeding does reduce fertility, it is still possible to conceive.

3 False. Yes you can get pregnant, so if you don't want to conceive straight away, take some precautions.

4 True. This is why unprotected sex, even before a woman ovulates, can result in pregnancy.

5 False. Yes you can, but if you are trying for a baby you increase your chances when penetration takes place.

Body MECHANICS!

You may not have done any biology since you left school, but now's the time to really find out about how your body works.

When thinking about having a baby a good starting point is to understand the mechanics or biology involved. By knowing some simple biology, you are more likely to make love at the optimum time and thus increase your chance of conceiving quickly. There are other benefits too, as if you are aware of what is going on inside you, and you know the medical terms, it can make a visit to the doctor, midwife or practice nurse seem less daunting.

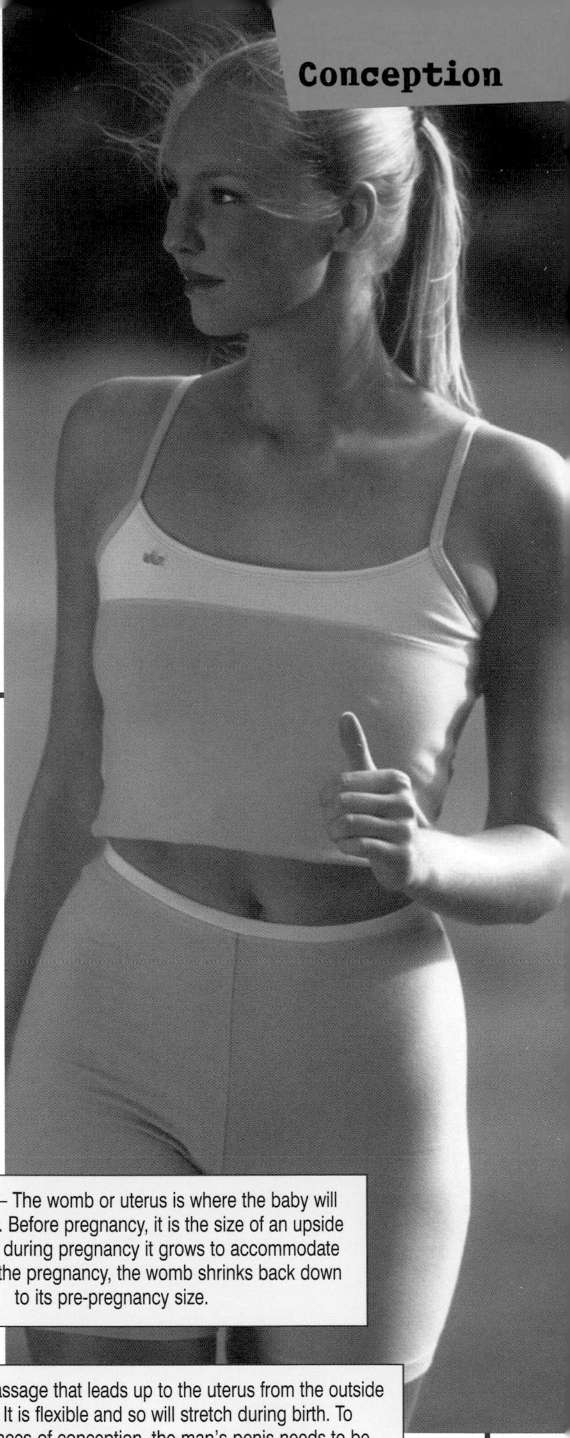

A quick tour of your anatomy

A good place to start is on the outside. While some women can label up parts of their external genitalia, do not worry if you are one of those who cannot. Don't worry either if parts of your genitalia appear larger or smaller than in the diagram. As with other body parts such as noses, ears and hands, genitalia come in many different sizes.

On the inside

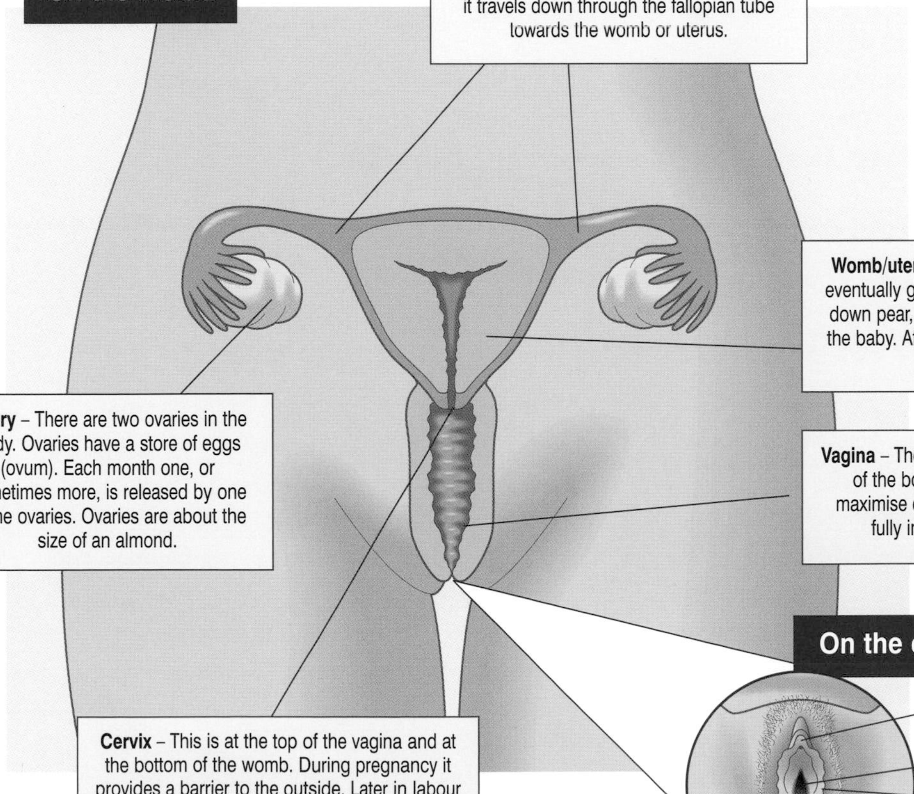

Fallopian tubes – Once the egg is released it travels down through the fallopian tube towards the womb or uterus.

Womb/uterus – The womb or uterus is where the baby will eventually grow. Before pregnancy, it is the size of an upside down pear, but during pregnancy it grows to accommodate the baby. After the pregnancy, the womb shrinks back down to its pre-pregnancy size.

Ovary – There are two ovaries in the body. Ovaries have a store of eggs (ovum). Each month one, or sometimes more, is released by one of the ovaries. Ovaries are about the size of an almond.

Vagina – The passage that leads up to the uterus from the outside of the body. It is flexible and so will stretch during birth. To maximise chances of conception, the man's penis needs to be fully inside the vagina when he ejaculates or 'comes'.

Cervix – This is at the top of the vagina and at the bottom of the womb. During pregnancy it provides a barrier to the outside. Later in labour it opens up to allow the baby to pass through and down into the vagina.

On the outside

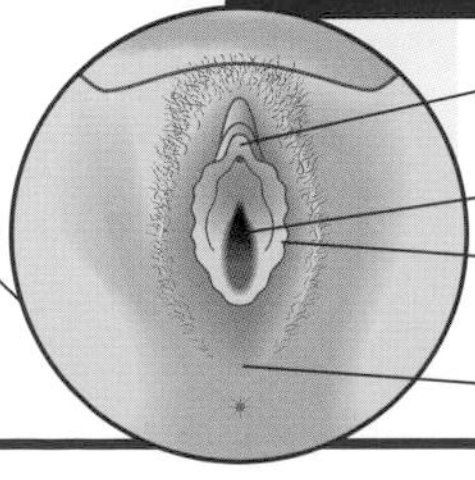

Clitoris

Opening of the vagina

Vulva

Perineum

how the menstrual cycle works

THE MENSTRUAL CYCLE PROVIDES US WITH ONE OF THE KEYS AS TO PREDICTING A WOMAN'S FERTILE TIMES. THE MENSTRUAL CYCLE CAN BE DIVIDED INTO THREE KEY PHASES:

Phase 1

FROM MENSTRUATION TO OVULATION

This phase begins after your period. During this phase the lining of the uterus is prepared and the egg becomes ready. The length of this phase varies between women. In some women this phase may last 18 or more days, while for others it is only 12 or even less. Some women also find that one month they can have quite a long phase and then another time have a much shorter phase. It is important to find out the length of your own phase (see p.16) and to see if there is a pattern to it. Making love in the last part of this phase means that sperm will be available to fertilise the egg. This means that you can increase your chances of conceiving if you have sex in the five days leading up to ovulation.

Phase 2

OVULATION

The egg is released from one of the ovaries. Women are fertile in this phase, although it is fairly short as the egg needs to be fertilised within two to three days.

Phase 3

MENSTRUATION (HAVING A PERIOD)

In this phase, the lining of the womb becomes thick enough to receive a fertilised egg. If the egg has not been fertilised, the lining is shed and preparation begins again ready for the next cycle. The unused lining disintegrates and passes down through the neck of the womb and out through the vagina. This is a woman's monthly bleed or period.

Did you know

Only three out of every twenty-five women will have an 'average' 28 day cycle.

Contrary to popular belief, the ovaries do not take it in turns each month to release the egg. There appears to be no particular pattern.

An egg can be fertilised for between two to three days after ovulation.

Over to the men!

It takes two to make a baby and so now is a good time for both of you to know how men's bodies work. As with other body parts, the size of a man's penis varies. Contrary to popular belief, the size of a man's penis does not make any difference to their ability to make a woman pregnant.

Production of sperm

It is worth understanding that sperm production is important. Failure to conceive is sometimes the result of a low sperm count. Men produce sperm in their testes. It takes 100 days for sperm to be ready for their eventual journey. For optimum production of sperm, the testes need to be kept cooler than the rest of the body. Normally body temperature is 37.2°C, but the scrotum ensures that the testes are kept between 2°C and 5°C lower.

Studies have found that the wearing of tight fitting underwear, trousers and shorts can reduce significantly the number of sperm a man produces. This is because the testes are being kept too close to the body and air cannot circulate around to cool them off. In the same way, men who sit down for long periods can also have a lower sperm count. Hot baths and showers can also have the same effect! Sperm production can also be affected by other factors such as diet, excessive alcohol, smoking and exercise.

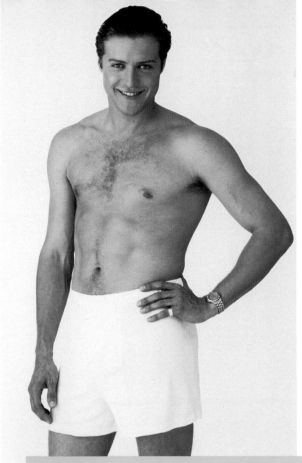

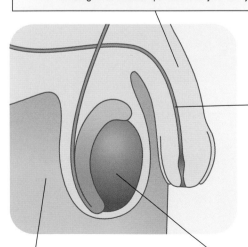

Penis – The penis is made of a special tissue, which fills with blood when the man becomes aroused. This causes the penis to gradually become harder and then erect. During sex, sperm travels from the testes via a tube called the 'vas deferens', along the urethra in the penis to be ejaculated. Ideally, ejaculation needs to take place in the woman's vagina so that the sperm can carry on their journey.

Urethra – The tube that runs down through the penis. When a man ejaculates, sperm travels down the urethra. The urethra is also used to carry urine from the bladder, although both these functions do not happen at the same time!

Scrotum – This is the bag of skin that is directly under the penis and contains the testes or 'balls'. The scrotum protects the testes, but more importantly keeps them at a constant cool temperature, which is below body temperature.

Testes – There are two testes which feel ball-like hence the expression 'balls'. Sperm is made and stored in the testes.

Did you know

A batch of sperm takes 100 days to produce.

Men who wear tight trousers and underwear produce less fertile sperm.

Up to 300 million sperm are produced when a man ejaculates.

Only 50–100 sperm will reach the fallopian tubes.

Sperm capable of fertilising an egg can live for up to five days.

The journey towards
conception

1 When a man ejaculates or 'comes' into a woman's vagina, the sperm begin their amazing journey. Some sperm leak out of the vagina but others will find their way through the cervix. The speed at which the sperm can swim partly depends on the mucus in the woman's cervix. At the time around ovulation, it is quite thin and plentiful and this allows the sperm to move easily through it.

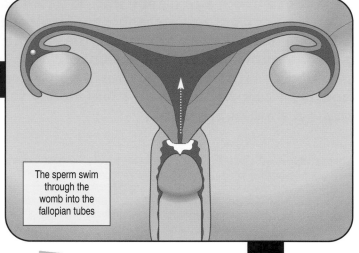

The sperm swim through the womb into the fallopian tubes

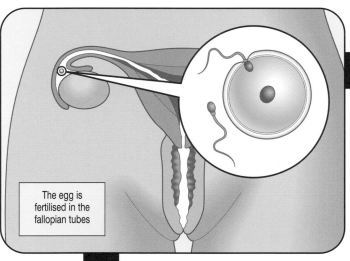

The egg is fertilised in the fallopian tubes

2 The sperm swim along through the womb and into the fallopian tubes. Some do not survive the journey. Conception takes place when one sperm meets up and joins with a newly-released egg. If sex has taken place just before ovulation, the sperm will be waiting, while if sex takes place on or the day after ovulation, the sperm will catch up with the egg as it reaches the top of the fallopian tube. If sex takes place a few days after ovulation, the egg will have already deteriorated and so it unlikely that fertilisation, which will result in a pregnancy, will take place.

3 Following conception, the fertilised egg or embryo travels down the fallopian tube and into the womb. It is already beginning to grow and the womb is ready to receive it. The embryo attaches itself to the lining of the womb. Hormones are released which stop the shedding of the lining of the womb. This means that a woman misses her period.

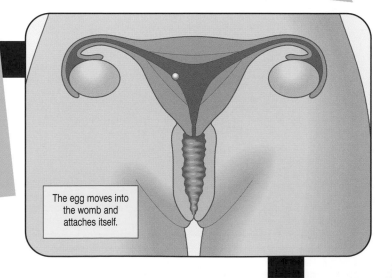

The egg moves into the womb and attaches itself.

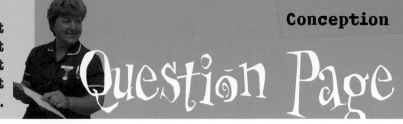

While it is easy to find out information about pregnancy, finding out about how to conceive is not always so easy. **Verity Hardy, senior midwife,** looks at some of the common questions that women ask about getting pregnant.

Question Page

Q I have heard that you should start taking folic acid before you get pregnant. Is this true and will it help me to conceive?

A Vitamins and minerals such as folic acid play appear to have an enormous impact on our overall health. The full significance of deficiencies is not at present known but we do know that diet and nutrition have an effect on our ability to conceive and maintain a healthy pregnancy. Folic acid supplements have been shown to dramatically cut down the risk of having a baby with spina bifida or neural tube defects. This is why women are advised to take a 400 mcg supplement while they are trying to get pregnant and also during the first twelve weeks of their pregnancy. If you are already pregnant, you should take folic acid as soon as you find out.

Q I have very irregular periods. Will this mean that I will take longer to conceive?

A Many women have irregular periods and still find that they can conceive in a short space of time. In some cases conception may take a little longer as you may not ovulate very frequently. This means that it can be useful to know when you are at your most fertile. Consider keeping a diary of your periods because you may find that even though your periods are irregular, there is still some sort of pattern to them. You may also find it helpful to keep a note of changes to your cervical fluid and temperature as these can be good predictors of when you are about to ovulate.

Q My mother is a non-identical twin and I am wondering if there is a chance that I will conceive twins?

A Identical twins are created when a fertilised egg divides into two. Non-identical twins are the result of two eggs being released and being separately fertilised. Twins can run in families following the maternal line. Because your mother was a twin, this means that there is a slightly higher chance that you may conceive twins. Overall, women have a 1 in 80 chance of naturally conceiving twins.

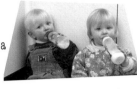

Q I am 35 years old. Have I left it too late?

A Fertility is dependent upon a number of factors. It is true that fertility does decline in age, but there are many women of your age and older who do conceive. Try and make sure that your diet and lifestyle is healthy and make sure that your partner is also looking after himself (see p.16).

Q I have epilepsy. How will this affect my chances of conception?

A You will be pleased to hear that epilepsy should not affect your ability to conceive and have a healthy baby. You should however make an appointment to visit the doctor before you try for a baby. This is important because your doctor will need to review any prescribed medication that you are taking in case it may affect the development of the baby.

Q When is the best time of the month to try for a baby?

A You actually increase your chances of conceiving if you have sex during the two or three days before your ovary releases an egg or on the day you ovulate. This is because the sperm can survive and be fertile for up to five days and the egg may be fertilised for up to two days after ovulation. So this gives the maximum time for fertilisation to take place. The danger of waiting until after ovulation is that if your body decides to ovulate a day or so earlier than you expected the sperm may miss their opportunity! As women's cycles can vary, try to learn about yours.

Q I have been told that it is better to remain flat after we have made love.

A There are many anecdotal stories about how best to conceive. Staying flat, putting a cushion underneath you or keeping your partner inside you after he has ejaculated are common tips. At the end of the day, there is currently no research that either proves or disproves these ideas. This means that it is completely up to you as to whether you wish to try this one out. You should however try to make sure that your partner ejaculates fully into your vagina as this does increase the likelihood of conception. Aim also to have sex around the time you ovulate.

While the average menstrual cycle is about 28 days, not all women are 'average'!

In order to maximise your chances of getting pregnant it is helpful to understand a bit more about your menstrual cycle so you know when your most fertile period is likely to be. The average menstrual cycle is 28 days but for many women this is not the case.

Follow the steps on these pages to help you learn more about your cycle and understand when you are at your most fertile and most likely to conceive.

Getting a feel for your cycle length

1 Put the start date of your period on the calendar.

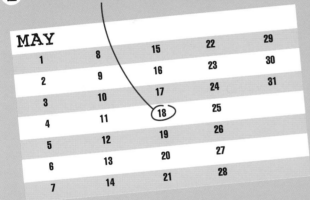

2 Next time you have a period, write the start date on the calendar.

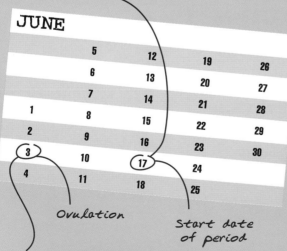

Ovulation

Start date of period

3 Count back 14 days to find the approximate date of your ovulation. You can now begin to get a feel of the length of the first phase of your cycle which leads up to ovulation.

4 This is the phase that can vary between women. In this example the length of the first phase is 16 days.

5 To get a real picture of your cycle, it is a good idea to track in this way for several more periods.

Noting down other changes in your body

As well as using a diary method to learn about your menstrual cycle, some women find it useful to notice the way that their cervical fluid changes. The cervix secretes mucus throughout the menstrual cycle, but the mucus changes at different points in the cycle. Around ovulation, it increases and becomes much thinner, slippery and stretchy. If you were to put some between your finger and thumb, you would find that it would stretch several centimetres. It is often compared to raw egg white. This mucus is designed to help the sperm swim easily through it and nourish it. This is a good indicator that you are in your fertile phase. This is the time to have sex if you want to get pregnant, or to use contraception if you do not! A few days after ovulation, the mucus changes again. This time there is less of it and it is thick and cloudy. In this state it is hostile to sperm.

> The best time to make love if you want a baby is at the end of the first phase of your menstrual cycle, just before you ovulate. Look out for thin, stretchy and clear cervical mucus as a sign that you are about to ovulate. If you have been taking your temperature each day when you first wake up, you should see a small drop followed by a rise.

Temperature

Another way in which you could find out about your menstrual cycle is by keeping a note of your temperature each morning just after you wake up. Your temperature changes at different points in the cycle, dropping just before you ovulate and then rising when ovulation has taken place. Tracking your temperature means that you can work out when you are most likely to become pregnant. This is a particularly good method to use if your cycles are really irregular.

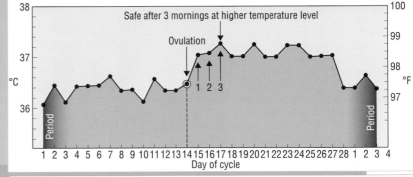

Taking your temperature

Tracking your temperature is quite easy, although you will need to be quite organised. You should have everything to hand as the idea is that you take your temperature when you first wake up. This means that the body is at rest and gives you what is known as you basal body temperature (BBT). You will need an accurate thermometer and a piece of paper to note down the results.

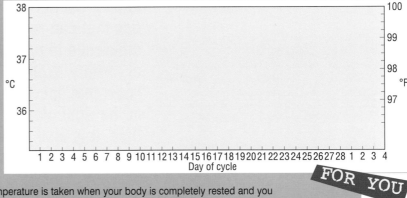

1 Pop the thermometer under your tongue for two or three minutes when you first wake up. You must do this every day to get an accurate picture.

2 Avoid having anything to drink or eat – the idea is that your temperature is taken when your body is completely rested and you have not had the time to rush around.

3 Make a note of the results. You could plot them on the blank chart that we have provided.

4 Look to see when your temperature is falling and then begins to rise again.

5 This pattern indicates first of all that you are about to ovulate and when it rises that you are ovulating.

Using ovulation kits

Some women use ovulation predictor kits to help them predict their fertile phase. Ovulation predictor kits are available from chemists and are reasonably reliable and fairly simple to use. They work by detecting a hormone in your urine that increases when ovulation is about to take place. Ovulation kits are not able to tell you exactly when the egg is about to released, but will be able to predict that you will ovulate between 12-36 hours after a positive result. You may have to keep repeating the tests on different days to find out when you are most likely to ovulate. While some couples find that ovulation predictor kits are very helpful, others find that they can create tension and it make sex feel very clinical.

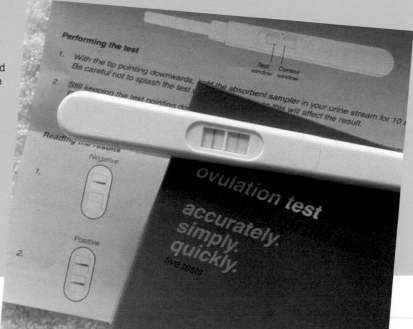

Top tips

TO HELP CONCEPTION

Conception can be a bit of lottery, but here are some tips that can really make a difference to both your levels of fertility. While most people know that sperm need to be in the right place at the right time, it is also important for both of your bodies to be providing the right conditions.

Eat a healthy balanced diet

Food is amazingly important. The body needs vitamins and minerals that are found in a range of foods to provide it with the chemicals it needs to produce healthy sperm, eggs and also to provide the lining in the womb. If you have been on the pill for a long time you may be low on certain vitamins and minerals, especially vitamin B complexes. This means that you might consider checking up on your diet (see p.28) Women should also take a 400 mcg folic acid tablet as part of their daily diet as this can prevent spina bifida and neural tube defects.

Avoid alcohol

It is a good idea for you both to avoid alcohol or at least to really cut down. There are many reasons for this, but the key is to remember that however much you like a drink, it does act as a poison in the body. It lowers men's sperm count even when men are only drinking small amounts. It also prevents the body from taking in those essential minerals and vitamins that are needed for conception. Finally, it is worth knowing that as well as potentially causing damage to unborn babies, it can also cause miscarriages.

Give up smoking

Just like alcohol, smoking is another poison for the body. There is plenty of research to show that both men's and women's levels of fertility drop when you smoke. Sadly, smoking also causes babies to be born prematurely and this affects their long-term health and even ability to survive.

Take some gentle, regular exercise

Exercise has many benefits and can help to reduce stress as well as stimulate some essential hormones. You should both, however, avoid excessive fitness regimes as these can actually reduce your levels of fertility.

Keep sperm count up by wearing cotton boxer shorts and avoiding hot baths

A common cause of low sperm count in men is simply down to the testes being overheated. This means that you should avoid tight fitting underwear, lycra shorts and having hot baths and showers. You should also avoid sitting down for long periods as this can reduce your fertility. Choose boxer shorts made if possible out of cotton. As it takes up to six months to improve sperm count, you should keep up this regime until conception has taken place.

MEN ONLY

Get to know your cycle and work out when you are likely to ovulate

If you take the time to work out when your body releases the egg during your cycle, you will start to get an idea of when you should be making love. (see p.16)

WOMEN ONLY

Enjoy each other's company and find time to do things together

It is not unusual for couples to find baby making stressful. It can quickly become clinical and this in turn is likely to have some effect on your ability to conceive. Spending time together and enjoying yourselves can reduce any stress. It's not perhaps surprising that many couples who go away on holiday, having decided not to bother with baby making for a while, return only to find that a pregnancy has been achieved.

Have sex around the time that you ovulate

As conception is about sperm being in the right place at the right time, you can maximise your chances of conception by making love when you are at your most fertile.

Avoid seeing 'baby making' as a race or competition

Stress can really affect conception. Although it can be disheartening to suddenly notice that everyone else seems to have a baby or young children, try not to see it as a race. Also consider additional stresses in your life, at work or home, as they may also reduce your chances of getting pregnant. Deal with these issues as best you can, take regular breaks from work and time out for yourself and your partner. Do think about visiting your GP, however, if you have not conceived after 12 months of trying. Take any useful information with you, like a temperature chart and your diary, so the doctor can see how your cycle works.

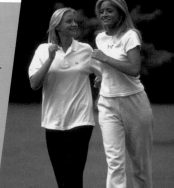

Boy or girl
can you help nature?

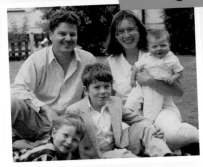

If nature is left to her own devices around 105 boys will be born for every 100 girls. But what if you are hoping for a boy or are particularly desperate for a girl. Can you improve on nature's odds?

Sex or gender selection has always been a hot topic. While it is possible for scientists and doctors to identify sperm and select sperm to create a child of a particular sex, this is only done under the strictest controls and for medical reasons. For example, doctors will help couples to have a girl if they know that otherwise a boy would develop a life-threatening condition such as muscular dystrophy.

For couples hoping to have a child of a particular sex, there are some ways in which you can improve on nature's odds, although you may still not beat nature.

A good starting point is to understand that a child's sex is the result of two chromosomes. One chromosome comes from each parent. A boy needs an X chromosome and a Y chromosome. A girl needs two separate X chromosomes.

Women's eggs automatically provide an X chromosome and so the lottery of sex selection revolves around a man's sperm. Half of a man's sperm will be carrying the Y chromosome and the other half the X chromosome. Sex selection therefore depends on which type of sperm fertilises the egg. A Y sperm that fertilises the egg will produce a boy (XY) while an X sperm will produce a girl (XX).

Scientists have noticed that there are differences between X sperm and Y sperm and tips to conceive a particular sex of children are based around these differences. Y sperm are faster, but tire more easily. They prefer alkaline conditions which are found higher in the vagina and are also created when a woman has an orgasm. X sperm are heavier and slightly slower swimmers, although they have greater stamina.

Caroline and her husband Stuart have three boys aged five, three and 14 months.

'I already had two boys and was really hoping for a girl. It seemed that among my friends everyone who wanted a boy got a girl and those of us who wanted girls got boys. Ideally, we were only going to have two children, but I was so hoping for a daughter we thought we would try one last time. I read up a bit and we tried to make sure that we had sex way before the time of ovulation. I had also read that diet can make a difference and so we were busy eating all sorts of foods. In the end though we had another boy. We found out at the scan because although I didn't want to know ahead, you could just tell by the pictures that it was a boy. I had a little cry by myself afterwards. I was crying for the daughter that I was never going to have. Just one day though, and then I went out and bought some really nice baby clothes for the little boy. When I gave birth, it didn't matter. It was so fantastic to have a new healthy baby. It was love at first sight and he is so very, very precious.'

Tips to conceive a girl
- Have frequent intercourse after menstruation to reduce the numbers of male sperm.
- Stop two or three days before ovulation.
- Do not have sex for a week after ovulation.

Tips to conceive a boy
- Avoid having sex in the days before ovulation.
- Try to ejaculate deep into the vagina.

Ann and her husband have three boys and a girl

'We had three boys and while I really wanted another baby, we both quite fancied a girl. I had read somewhere that if you have three of the same sex there is 75% chance of repeating the same sex. So I read up a bit and we did use the timing method. I would like to think that it did work for us, but we'll never really know if it was that or just because we got lucky. I think the thing though is to make sure that

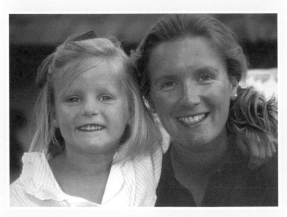

you really want a baby in the first place. Getting Fay was wonderful, but we would still have loved another boy. It's having a child that's the most important.'

Time *Waiting*

Deciding to start a family is a big step, but once the decision is taken, most people just want to know how long it will take. We talk to Annette Briley about how long it may take and also what you can do if no baby appears.

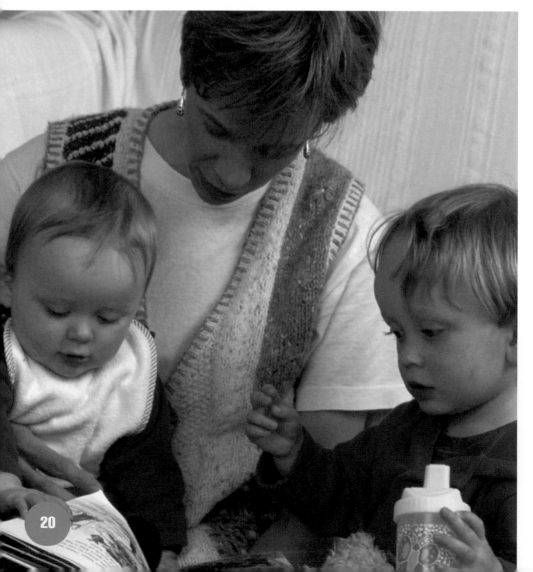

It would appear that conception is a bit of a lottery. Annette says, 'It varies enormously from person to person. Some women get pregnant straight away, but then it is not uncommon for others to take up to a year.' This is borne out by statistics which suggest that around 85% of couples will have managed to conceive a baby within a year. Annette suggests that it can be very hard to predict how quickly a woman will conceive as this is dependent on many factors and no couple will know just how fertile they are until they begin to try for their first child together. 'Managing to conceive the first child is often the hardest for most couples,' although she goes on to add that just because a woman has been fertile with one partner does not mean that she will automatically conceive when trying again in a new relationship. 'Sometimes a woman may have had no problem conceiving in one relationship, but with a new partner may have more difficulty. Equally, some women have found that conception with one partner proved difficult but with a new partner they conceived quite quickly'.

Getting caught out

While there are couples who may take a few months to conceive, a significant number of couples conceive in their first month. This can come as a shock to couples who believe that it always takes a few months before the women will get pregnant. Annette reminds couples that nature can play tricks and often women become pregnant when they least expect it. 'Some people are caught out, but if you stop using contraception and you desperately don't want a baby at a certain time, perhaps because you have a holiday booked, you should use condoms in this time.'

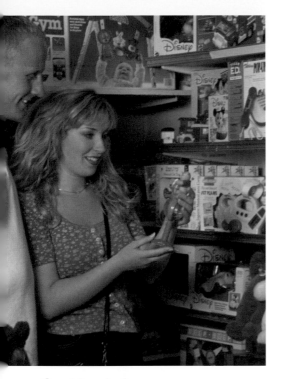

Seeking help

Many women are not sure how long they should wait before consulting their doctor if they have not conceived. 'We used to advise women to wait for a couple of years, but this has changed,' Annette explains. 'Waiting for such a time can be very stressful for couples and so we now feel that you should see your doctor when you are beginning to get worried and that it is taking over your life. For most women, this is often towards the end of their first year of trying.' A visit to the doctor can feel daunting but there are ways of preparing for the visit. Annette suggests that it is helpful if you have kept a diary of your periods or have an idea about your cycle. 'The doctor is likely to ask you about your menstrual cycle, the date of your last period and so the more information that you have the better. This will help the doctor make an initial assessment.' Nowadays many women choose to have their first babies later and often question how long they should wait if they have not conceived. Annette says, 'Women can get pregnant into their forties, but age does affect fertility and women who are older often feel a bit more under pressure as their body clock is ticking. It may be helpful for them to consult a doctor earlier rather than later if they have concerns.'

Annette is also keen to remind women that while they are waiting to conceive, there are positive things that they can do in order to boost their chances not only of conception, but also of having a healthy baby. 'Women should try and get themselves into good physical shape, eat well and also to cut down on smoking and alcohol. It is important that they check with their doctor whether or not they need a rubella (German measles) injection. Contracting rubella in pregnancy can cause problems for the unborn child.'

Real lives

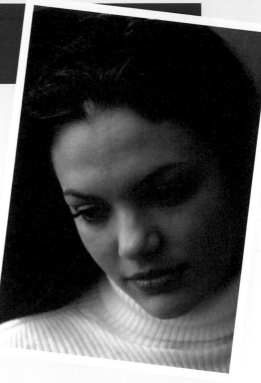

Laura and Gary now have two children, Rory and Sara, but as Laura explains getting pregnant the first time wasn't that easy.

I was 33 when I first started trying for a baby. Gary and I got married and we thought that we would have the first year just for ourselves. The following year we started trying. I thought that I might get caught straight away, but it didn't work out that way. After a few months, I began to get really disheartened. I was a bit older than some of my friends and they all seemed to be pushing out babies, left right and centre. Several times I did tests thinking that I was pregnant, but each time it was negative and I would think no, not this month and on it went. I did feel quite lonely as I had lost my mum and although I had really good friends, I just couldn't really tell them what I was feeling. I know that I put on a really bright face but actually there were days at one point when I couldn't face going into town. Suddenly it seemed that there were babies everywhere. All these women had prams and toddlers and I was the only one who didn't have a pushchair. Gary was great, he kept on saying that our time would come, but I know that inside he was a bit worried too. It seems silly now but I was so desperate for a baby that I was ready to try anything. When one friend mentioned that doing a handstand afterwards might work I even tried that.

It was nearly two years after we first started trying that my GP suggested that I should start out on fertility treatment. Gary was tested, but his sperm count was fine. I think that he was pleased about that, but it made me feel even worse. I thought then that it was my fault. The daft thing was that it was while I was waiting for my appointment at the hospital that I fell pregnant. It was like my getting pregnant was about to be in the hands of other people and so I relaxed. Finding out I was pregnant was wonderful. I wanted everyone to know. I was so proud of myself. Even though I now have two children, my heart still goes out to women who are having difficulties because I have been there. All I can say is don't give up, but do learn about your body. I realise now that I never knew enough about my cycle partly because it was so irregular. With Sara, I checked my cervical mucus and so had some idea of when was a good time for us. I think that, and the fact that I was more relaxed, made a lot of difference. I fell pregnant with her after a couple of months.

Next PLEASE!

Having been through one pregnancy and birth, many people soon find that they are thinking about another. We look at some of the common questions that women ask when thinking about a further addition to their family.

Q How long should I wait before trying for another baby?

A Some people have their children very close together, while others choose to space them out. Only you and your partner can tell whether or not you are ready to cope with the demands of a new pregnancy. You might however think about your health and level of tiredness. Consider whether you are physically recovered from your previous pregnancy and labour. Pregnancy does put some stress on the body and so it is a good idea to get back in shape before starting again. Begin by taking folic acid supplements, thinking about your diet and overall level of fitness. If you have had any complications in the pregnancy or during the birth, it will be very important to see a doctor before conceiving so that your next pregnancy can be supported from the very start. You may be referred to an obstetrician very early in the next pregnancy.

Q Can I conceive while I am breastfeeding?

A While breastfeeding provides a wonderful start for your baby, some people think that it can also be used as contraception. This is not quite the case and although breastfeeding can reduce your fertility, you would be advised to use contraception if you are not intending to have another baby straight away. Breastfeeding in itself is not a reliable contraceptive. If you are hoping to become pregnant while breastfeeding, you may find that you have to wait for your periods to start again, as some women do not ovulate at all while they are breastfeeding. Your menstrual cycle is more likely to return once your baby has been weaned.

Q I developed pre-eclampsia in my last pregnancy. Will this be a problem again?

A Pre-eclampsia is a potentially serious condition. It affects around 4% of pregnant women with the onset and the severity of it varying between women. It often appears in women's first pregnancies without any real reason and so you may find that you will not have it in another pregnancy. However, as this cannot be guaranteed, you should go and see your doctor or midwife once you know that you are pregnant. This means that you will be able to receive medical advice and support from the very start of your pregnancy. You will also find that your pregnancy will be carefully monitored to check for any early signs of the condition reappearing.

Q I had terrible morning sickness with my first baby. Will this happen again?

A Morning sickness is a reaction to the hormones that the body is producing to maintain a pregnancy. For some women, the nausea and sickness can be constant while for others it is only very slight. It is called morning sickness because many women find that it affects them particularly first thing when they wake up. There is no real way of telling how you will be with another pregnancy. Some women who are very sick can find that they hardly feel anything with another pregnancy. On the other hand, some women who escaped nausea and sickness first time are surprised to find that it hits them second time round. If you are worried about how you will cope in another pregnancy, it may be a good idea to talk this through with your doctor before trying again. It may be reassuring to know that many women cope with morning sickness more easily in later pregnancies because they have learnt ways of dealing and coping with it.

Q Will I be able to conceive more quickly now?

A While most women find it easier to conceive after already having a child, this is not the case for everyone. Firstly, your body needs to be physically ready to conceive again. This can take longer for some women than others. You can help your body by gently exercising, eating a balanced diet, taking folic acid and also checking that you are resting enough. If after a few months, you are beginning to get anxious, consider talking to your doctor or family planning clinic who will then be able to give you further support and advice.

Q I had an emergency caesarean section last time. Will I be able to have an ordinary delivery with another baby?

A Many women who have had a caesarean section are able to have a vaginal delivery later, but this depends on several factors, such as the reason why a caesarean was needed in the first place. The best person to advise you is your obstetrician who will have access to your medical records. If you wish to discuss this with your obstetrician, begin by contacting your doctor's surgery. You may also find it helpful to know that in most areas there are local support groups for women who have had caesarean sections that are organised through the National Childbirth Trust (tel: 0870 770 3236).

Q My partner is keen to have another baby. The trouble is that I don't think that I could love another baby like I do my little boy.

A Giving birth is a dramatic process. Many women feel very strongly attached to their children. This is the nature of maternal feelings or attachment. Your love is very special and so it is normal that you should question whether or not you could feel the same again. Fortunately, this type of love is not rationed and so while many parents find that they have slightly different relationships with each of their children, the strength of love that they feel is the same for each child. The final decision as to whether or not you are ready for another child though must lie with you. Feeling pressurised into another pregnancy before you are emotionally ready is not a good idea and may end up putting your relationship under stress. In the meantime both of you can enjoy your little boy.

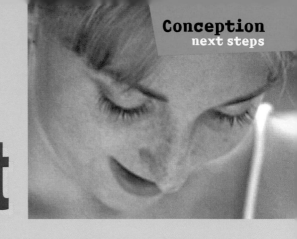

Finding out
that you are
pregnant

Ideally, it is best to know that you are pregnant as early on as possible. The first few weeks in a developing baby's life are crucial. Knowing that you are pregnant means that you can take extra care of yourself and your unborn child. So how can you tell if you are pregnant or not?

Changes to your body

When a woman becomes pregnant, the body begins to produce hormones in large quantities to maintain the pregnancy. These hormones result in many physical changes to the body. Women who have a multiple pregnancy, twins or triplets, are likely to have stronger physical signs in the early days due to higher levels of hormones. Some women say that they instinctively know that they are pregnant while others first realise when they begin to notice the physical changes to their bodies.

Missed period (amennorhoea)

One of the most reliable early signs that you may be pregnant is a missed period, especially if you have a regular cycle or have noted when you ovulate. Some women do not miss a period completely when they are first pregnant but instead have a very light period. If you have either missed a period or have had some very light periods, you may wish to consider taking a pregnancy test (see p.24).

Nausea and sickness (morning sickness)

The term 'morning sickness' is often used, but is misleading as women can feel nauseous and even be sick at any or several points in the day. Most, but not all women find that these feelings usually pass after the first twelve weeks or so.

Tiredness

It is common for women to feel very tired, drowsy and even irritable in the first few weeks of pregnancy.

Needing to pass water more often

Some women find that quite early on in their pregnancy they notice that they have to go to the toilet more often to pass water. This is caused by the womb beginning to grow and pressing down on the bladder.

Strong sense of smell and noticing a strange taste in the mouth

Many women find that they have a heightened sense of smell and notice particular dislike of odours such as fruit, petrol and cigarette smoke. Other women report a strange 'metallic' taste in their mouths. It is also common to find that women become hungrier or have particular food cravings.

Changes to breasts

One effect of the increased hormones is a change to the breasts. Many women notice that their breasts can feel larger and more tender. They may also tingle and the nipples may seem darker.

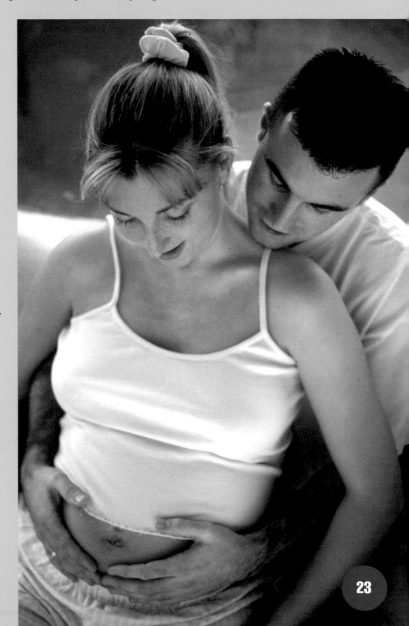

23

Some tell-tale signs of PREGNANCY

- **A missed period**

- **Feeling nauseous and even being sick, especially in the morning, although can be at any time**

- **A strong sense of smell**

- **Feelings of tiredness and irritability**

- **A metallic taste in the mouth**

- **Tender and slightly larger breasts than usual**

- **Needing to pee more often**

Pregnancy tests

Once you think that you are pregnant, it is important to confirm your suspicions with a pregnancy test. Pregnancy tests work by detecting a hormone called human chorionic gonadotrophin (HCG) in the urine. This is only made when a woman is pregnant and traces of it can be found in the urine from three days after conception. As the concentration of HCG continues to build up in the urine, most tests are carried out after women have missed a period. Doing a pregnancy test very early on can sometimes give a negative result because the levels of HCG may be too low for the test to pick up on. HCG can also be detected by blood tests, but most women provide a urine sample because it is easier.

Collecting a urine sample

The best time to collect a urine sample is first thing in the morning. This is because levels of HCG will have built up overnight. It is important to use a clean container. If you have washed something out, make sure that you rinse it well and allow for it to dry. A plastic or glass jar is the best.

Where can you go for tests?

Pregnancy tests can be done at your local chemist, doctor or family planning clinic either free of charge or for a small fee, although there may be a small delay. These tests have the advantage of being very accurate, and also very quick. If the urine sample is tested on the spot, you probably will be given the result after twenty minutes or so.

Home pregnancy test kits

Many women choose to do a home pregnancy test so that they can test in private and find out the result after a few minutes. The tests are considered to be quite accurate, although it is essential that you follow carefully the manufacturer's instructions. Choose a kit that you think will be easy for you to use and make sure that you understand what mark or symbol will appear if the test is positive.

Some kits allow you to test yourself on the first day of your missed period. If you do decide to test at this point, do

not assume that a negative result will be always accurate. Levels of HCG in the very early days of pregnancy may not be sufficient for a home test to pick up, and so you might need to carry out a further test. If, however, you have obtained a positive result, this is generally very reliable.

The results of the test

While a positive result is likely to be accurate, a negative result may be misleading. It is not uncommon for women to have a negative result and to test again a week later and find that it is positive. This is because the levels of HCG gradually build up and may not be detected early on. If you test yourself very early on and you have a negative result, it is always wise to carry out another test if you still have not had a period. If you continue to get negative results and still no period, you should consult your doctor.

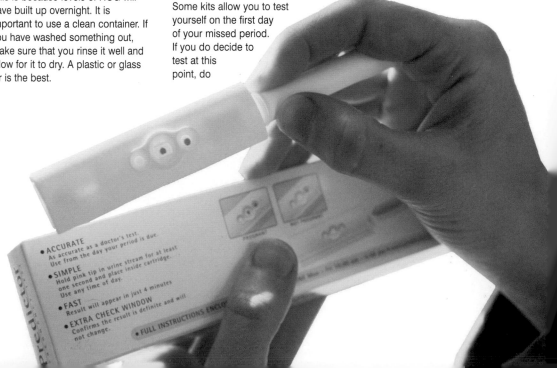

next steps

SO YOU'VE JUST FOUND OUT YOU ARE PREGNANT. WHAT SHOULD YOU DO NEXT? WHO SHOULD YOU TELL? WE ANSWER SOME OF YOUR QUESTIONS

Q When should I go and see my doctor?

A Most women choose to go and see their doctor quite quickly after they have had a pregnancy test. The advantage of going to see your doctor is that you will be given advice and support right from the start. Your doctor is likely to take your blood pressure, weigh and measure you and also tell you about the antenatal (pre-birth) services in your local area. The other advantage of going to the doctor early is that you will be given a form that you can send away to get free prescriptions and dental care.

Q How common is it to have a miscarriage and is there anything I can do to stop it happening to me?

A Sadly, miscarriages are quite common. It is thought that one in five pregnancies may end in miscarriage. But as the majority occur in the first twelve weeks or so, some women may not even know that they had been pregnant. Happily, the majority of women who have a miscarriage go on to have successful pregnancies. In terms of preventing a miscarriage, there is very little that you can do, although it is important to stop smoking, drinking alcohol and using recreational drugs. You should also rest and eat sensibly. If you have already had more than one pregnancy that has ended in miscarriage, talk to your doctor.

Q Can my employer give me the sack if I am pregnant?

A Definitely not! You have exactly the same rights to employment as before and your employer cannot use your pregnancy as an excuse to sack you. It is against the law for your employer to treat you unfairly. Your employer must also give you time off to attend antenatal clinics and check ups. Later on in your pregnancy, you will also be entitled to paid maternity leave and after the baby is born your job must be kept for you. Your employer may ask you for confirmation that you are pregnant. A good source of free advice about your rights is your local Citizens Advice Bureau. Their number will be in your local telephone directory.

Q I am unemployed and now pregnant. Will I get any help?

A Yes, there are several benefits that you can claim. As the benefits system can be quite complicated, the best thing to do is to go and visit your local benefits office or visit your local Citizens Advice Bureau. Don't be afraid of asking for help with form-filling or taking a friend along with you.

Q I think I got pregnant on a night when I was very drunk. How will this affect the baby?

A Firstly, you should stop worrying, as it is not possible to put the clock back and stress can have a harmful effect on your baby. You should now try to avoid alcohol especially if you are still in the first twelve weeks of your pregnancy. As your baby's development will be assessed using ultrasound scanning, you will soon be able to get further reassurance.

Q I am ten weeks pregnant and have a skiing holiday booked in a few weeks' time. Is it still safe to go?

A While the advice for pregnant women is to carry on with their normal activities including sports, it is always wise to be sensible. If you are a first time skier or have not skied in a long time, it may be useful to seek some advice from your doctor or midwife. You should also look at the terms of your holiday insurance to check that you will be covered while pregnant for any medical expenses that you may incur.

The Essential Early pregnancy checklist

- Make an appointment to see your doctor ☐
- Do not take any medication unless prescribed by your doctor ☐
- Carry on or start taking 400mcg folic acid supplement a day ☐
- Check to see whether you have had a rubella injection or are rubella immune ☐
- Eat a balanced diet which includes five portions of fruit and vegetables a day ☐
- Avoid liver, soft cheese, uncooked eggs such as boiled eggs, shellfish, and undercooked or cured meats ☐
- Wash all fruit and vegetables carefully, including pre-packed salads ☐
- Avoid drinking any alcohol especially in the first twelve weeks ☐
- Do not use any recreational or street drugs – get help if this is hard for you (see p. 48) ☐
- Give up smoking if you can, or at least cut right down ☐
- Avoid changing cats' litter tray or wear gloves and wash hands afterwards ☐
- Use gloves if doing any gardening ☐
- Rest when you feel tired or sick. ☐

Ante Natal Clinic

pause for THOUGHT

So what's it like to find out you're pregnant?

Pregnancy whether planned or not can create a whole new set of emotions. While some women are immediately over the moon, it is not uncommon for others to feel scared and quite unsure about the whole thing even when the pregnancy has been planned. Wendy Lidgate, a Health Visitor, explains that this is completely normal and that there are many reasons behind it. 'Pregnancy unleashes a huge range of emotions and thoughts. Women may be worried about how their partners will react and how the pregnancy is going to affect their relationship. It is also common for women to think about how well they will cope with being a parent as it can seem like a huge leap into the unknown.'

❛It felt that someone was playing a bad joke on us❜

Many women report feelings of numbness and shock when they first find out that they are pregnant. Katie, mother to Oliver aged 12 months, remembers vividly the day she did her pregnancy test. 'We had been trying for a baby for over a year and the stress had become too much. In the autumn, we decided to move to a bigger house and forget about trying for a family. I found out I was pregnant the day after we had exchanged contracts. I couldn't believe it when this blue line appeared. It felt that someone was playing a bad joke on us as we had just committed ourselves to this huge mortgage which relied on my salary as well. I remember just sitting on the bed and trying to take it all in.'

❛It hit me that I would have to be responsible and grown up❜

Men too can find it hard to take in the news that their partners are pregnant. Tim explains how he felt 'I knew that Cathy really wanted a baby, but didn't really have any strong feelings either way to be honest. When she told me, I can't say that I felt that excited, although I was happy for her. I tried to sound pleased and I suppose that I was, but quite quickly it hit me that I would have to be responsible and grown up. I also began to think about whether I could be a good father and whether I could take this all on. It was also hard because Cathy didn't look any different and it was not until we went to the scan and I could see the baby that the idea of being a father really got me excited.'

❛I knew that I was pregnant, but didn't want to have to think about it❜

For women who have unplanned pregnancies, feelings can be even harder to manage as Zainab a single mother recalls, 'I knew that I was pregnant, but didn't want to have to think about it. I spent a couple of weeks, convincing myself that I wasn't, but knew that I should take the test. When it was positive, I put the strip in my drawer and tried not to think about it. I was scared to tell my boyfriend or my parents and just wanted it all to disappear. I felt that there was no one that I could really talk it through with. In the end, I blurted it out to my mum and she was alright about it, although my boyfriend stopped coming round.'

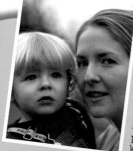

Rachel was 39 when she conceived Jack. She was not sure she wanted the baby as she explains.

I wasn't married or even intending to get pregnant and we were taking precautions. I think that I knew deep down that I was pregnant, but didn't want to think about it. I couldn't stop the thought though once my breasts began to tingle and my period had not come. I bought a home testing kit and did the test. I hadn't finished peeing on the strip when it changed to a definite blue. I had been expecting it. It was a jumble of feelings. My boyfriend was coming round anyway that evening so I just told him. He didn't want to know and said that I should have an abortion if we were going to be together. Next morning, I didn't want to discuss it with him. I felt quite alone, as I couldn't quite make my mind up what to do. In the end I made an appointment to see my GP. She was brilliant as I didn't really have anyone else I could to talk to and I knew my parents would be really shocked. She suggested that I start taking folic acid supplements even though I wasn't sure what I was going to do. A few days later, I had a slight bleed and got really worried. That made me realise that I wanted this baby and it might be my one and only chance to have a child. I was pushing forty and although financially secure, there was no real prospect of getting married. Fortunately, the bleed wasn't a miscarriage and can happen during pregnancy. After that, I just waited until I was over the twelve weeks mark and started to tell a few people. I hardly see my ex-boyfriend now and he is not interested in Jack. Once he had made his position clear, I knew that I would have to manage by myself.

My advice to other single women is not to worry about what people are going to say. In the end you've got to make your own decision and the right one for you. It was not like that at all. People were surprised, but really pleased for me, especially my family.

Being healthy before you try for a baby is incredibly important – not only do you give yourself the best chance of getting pregnant, but also you give your baby the best possible start in life.

We've got all the information for you here!

Whether it's finding out more about your ideal weight ...

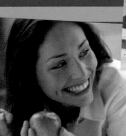

... or tips on how to achieve it – see the feature on our Three Step Plan.

Do you know what are the best ways if you want to lose weight? Check your knowledge with our quick quiz.

Fact or fiction

There are numerous myths about what foods are safe and what aren't when you're trying for a baby, are you right? Find out for yourself!

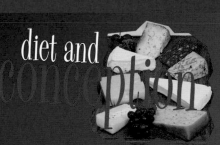

diet and conception

Many people know that they should be eating folic acid, but why? Do you know what can happen if you don't? Check out your knowledge.

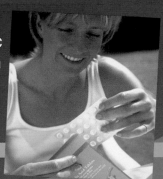

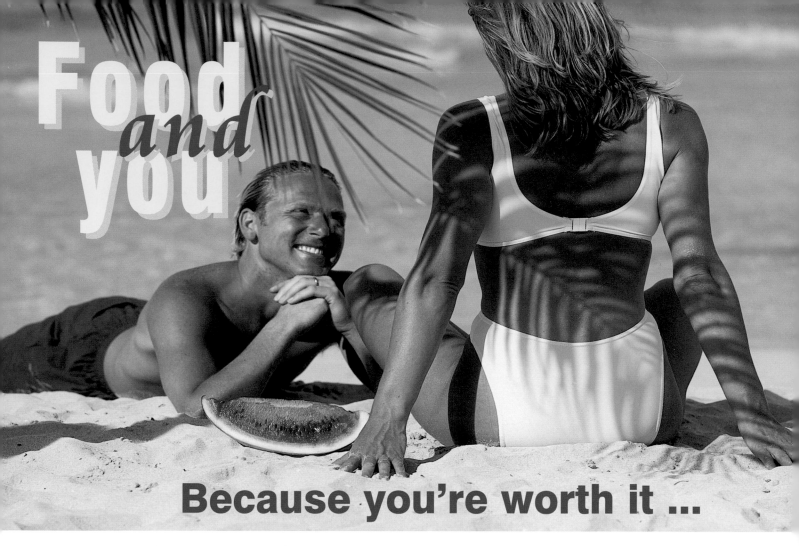

Food *and* you

Because you're worth it ...

Having a baby is one of life's great adventures. But being pregnant is also quite tiring. Aiming to be at the right weight for your build will not only help you through the pregnancy, but may also help you to conceive. We help you to work out your ideal weight and give you tips as to how to get there.

Being overweight or underweight is not ideal for conception or pregnancy. Pregnancy puts stress on the body and so being at the right weight gives your body quite an advantage. So how can you find out if you are at the right weight? There are several methods of checking your ideal weight, but many doctors and dieticians check a person's Body Mass Index (BMI). A score is given by working out a person's weight in relation to their height. Ideally your score should fall between 20 and 25.

WORKING OUT YOUR SCORE

You can either work out your score by looking at the chart below or having a go using a calculator. Either method is quite easy, although you will need to know your height in metres and your weight in kilos.

USING THE CHART

1 Find your height column along the bottom of the chart.

2 Now go upwards along the column until you can see your weight.

3 Look across to the very right now and see your body mass index score.

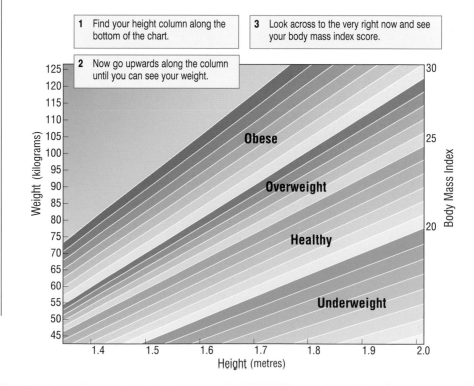

USING A CALCULATOR

You will need to know your height in metres and weight in kilograms.

Step 1 Write your height in each box and then multiply it. Write the answer in the total box.

Example

Height 1.58 x Height 1.58 = Total 2.496

Step 2 Put your weight in the first box and now divide it by the total from Step 1. This will give you body mass index score.

Example weight $61 Kg$ Divided by total from Step 1 2.496 = BMI 24.4

FOR YOU

Height ☐ x Height ☐ = Total ☐

FOR YOU

Example weight ☐ Divided by total from Step 1 ☐ = BMI ☐

SO HOW DID YOU DO?

YOUR BODY MASS INDEX SCORE IS UNDER 20

You are underweight. This means that you may find it harder to conceive and you may be lacking in nutrients. Think about switching to whole fat dairy products and also increase your calorie intake by adding oils, seeds, nuts and breads into your diet. If you do not have much of an appetite, consider eating several small meals a day and make sure that these are nutritious. If you are worried about your weight, make an appointment to see your GP.

YOUR BODY MASS INDEX SCORE IS BETWEEN 20 AND 25

Anywhere between these scores is considered to be fine. If you are at the top or lower ends of these scores, you may wish to keep an eye on your weight. You should still keep an eye on what you are eating and make sure that you are getting all the vitamins and minerals that your body needs.

YOUR BODY MASS INDEX SCORE IS BETWEEN 25 AND 30

If you are in this range, you might want to think about what you are eating and try to reduce your score. Look at our article 'A few pounds to spare' on p.31 for some tips and ideas.

YOUR BODY MASS INDEX SCORE IS OVER 30

For a really good start to conception, you should really think about reducing your scores. You may need some support and guidance. Consider making an appointment to see your doctor who may then be able to refer you to a dietician. You may also wish to consider joining a reputable slimming club. Choose one which will help you to lose weight gradually.

The BIG ISSUE

Five reasons why you should be at your ideal weight

1 BECAUSE YOU'RE WORTH IT
Being at or close to your ideal weight will make you feel healthy and look good. It will also make it easier for your body to cope with pregnancy and getting back into shape after the birth.

2 BECAUSE YOUR BABY IS WORTH IT
Research shows that women who are at their ideal weight are more likely to be able to carry the baby to the end of the pregnancy and that your baby will be a good weight when born. What you eat before and during pregnancy makes a real difference to the overall health and even intelligence of your baby.

3 BECAUSE YOU WILL CONCEIVE MORE EASILY
If you are very underweight or overweight, your fertility levels may be reduced.

4 BECAUSE YOU WILL HAVE AN EASIER PREGNANCY
Women who are at their ideal weight tend to have fewer complications during their pregnancies.

5 BECAUSE YOU ARE LIKELY TO HAVE AN EASIER BIRTH
Overweight women tend to have much larger babies. This can cause difficulties at birth.

! AND A BONUS POINT
Your good food habits will be passed on to future generations who will thank you!

Food and you:
LOVE OR HATE?

For most people, food is not just something that their bodies need to be supplied with. It's much more complicated than that as we all have a relationship with food and we eat for many reasons.
This relationship often begins in childhood. Taking a moment to think about your attitudes towards food is probably a good idea if you are trying to lose weight. It may mean that you will find it easier to change your eating patterns. It also has huge long-term benefits for your future children as your food habits and attitudes will rub off on them.

Do you always clear your plate even if you are full?

This habit is often learnt in childhood. Parents often praise children for eating everything up or get cross with them if something is left. You may have learnt that eating is about being 'good'. You may also not have learnt how to eat according to your appetite and so find that you eat even when you are not hungry. You may also find it hard to say 'no' to others who offer you food.

- Try using a smaller plate.
- Try leaving a little bit on the plate to break the habit.
- Practise saying 'no' to offers of food if you are not hungry.

With your own children try letting them serve themselves so that they can learn to judge their appetite. **FUTURE GENERATIONS**

Do you 'treat' yourself to sweet foods?

Sweets, chocolates and even puddings have traditionally been used as rewards for good behaviour by parents. Often parents say things such as, 'You're not allowed pudding until you have cleared your plate.' This means that sweet foods are often associated with pleasure, rewards and feelings of being good. It also means that people use food to treat themselves or comfort themselves.

- Instead of treating yourself with food, look for something else that you wouldn't normally buy, for example, a magazine or a favourite shower gel.
- If you still find that you need food to act as a treat, choose favourite fruits like strawberries or cherries, or pre-packed fruit salads.
- Help yourself to seconds of a main meal and see if you can break the habit of always having a pudding or dessert.

With your own children, try not to use food as rewards. If you want to treat children, give them crayons, a book or a container of bubble mix. **FUTURE GENERATIONS**

Do you think all foods are fattening?

Food can quickly become a huge obsession especially if you decide to go on a very strict diet. Sometimes, children learn from their parents that food is in some way 'bad' and this can lead to them wanting to diet from an early age. The truth is that food taken in the right amounts will not make you fat. It will keep you healthy and allow your body to function properly. This means that it is perfectly normal to enjoy your food and take pleasure in eating it.

- Enjoy your food.
- Make sure that you are eating at least five portions of fruit and vegetables a day.
- Eat cakes, biscuits, ice creams and other foods that are high in fat from time to time. You do not need to cut them out completely.

Do you have to eat when watching T.V?

The trouble with eating in front of the television is that you go into 'automatic' mode. You may find that you eat far more than you intended simply because you were just munching away without noticing it. Watching television is also quite passive. Your hands are likely to be free and so eating gives you something to do. Adverts on television can also make us feel hungry.

- Go out of the room when food adverts come on.
- Try doing something else while watching television. You could take up knitting or do the ironing.
- If you really need to chew or eat, try chewing gum or buy foods that are a bit fiddly to eat, for example, nuts that you have to crack open.
- Cut down on the amount of television you are watching – go out for a walk with your partner, spend time cooking great meals. Once your baby arrives, time for watching TV may well be reduced!

With your own children, get them into the habit of eating at the table so that they do not associate watching television with eating. **FUTURE GENERATIONS**

Do you find that you eat when you are bored or when you are alone?

Humans are actually designed to be active. When we are bored, the brain looks for ways of being stimulated. Eating is a very sensory experience and so stimulates the brain. This is why some people find that they turn to food when they are alone or are bored. Interestingly, people who have varied interests and who are busy can find it easier to lose weight.

- Identify times when you are most likely to be bored and try to change what you are doing.
- If you are bored at work, think about looking out for something more challenging or look out for some training.
- Take up a new hobby or activity.

With your own children, make sure that they are active, have friends and enjoy doing lots of different things. **FUTURE GENERATIONS**

a few pounds to spare?

So you want to lose weight before you get pregnant.. There are so many products and diets around, so what is the best way of losing, and more importantly keeping off those unwanted pounds? We ask our nutritional expert, Sarah Fulton, for some advice.

Sarah's first message to all would-be parents is that they have chosen a fantastic moment to think about their diet and their health. 'It's an ideal time to lose weight because it's about lifestyle change. It really is a golden opportunity to learn good life style habits so that they can be passed onto your child.'

"Diets are not appropriate for 99% of people"

Like most food experts, Sarah doesn't like the idea of restrictive fad diets. She explains, 'A diet is temporary, while what you need to do is adopt a permanent change of life. Diets are not appropriate for 99% of people.' She goes onto explain, 'Many people will have friends who swear by this and that diet and it starts off all marvellous. But go back and see the same people in six months time. Have they kept the weight off?'

This is because diets do not really work. As Sarah explains, 'They are often too restrictive and end up with people finding that they cannot keep them up. They end up breaking them, losing control and eating everything in sight. This makes them feel guilty, which is sad because food should be enjoyable.' She goes on to explain that diets also confuse the body and women who repeatedly diet are more likely to end up heavier 'the reasons why diets don't work are quite complex. Going on a fad diet slows down the metabolic rate and so when you eat again, the body finds it hard to use up the energy and puts it down as fat.' Sarah goes on to caution women who are following a strict diet when trying to conceive. 'Strict dieting, especially if

it means cutting out whole food groups such as dairy products or carbohydrates, can be very damaging. Women run the risk of depriving their bodies of essential nutrients.'

"Women who are pregnant should not be dieting"

Sarah also has a strong message for women who are already pregnant and want to lose weight. 'It's absolutely wrong for women who are pregnant to

try and follow a diet. Actively trying to lose weight in pregnancy may result in the baby not getting enough nutrients.' Sarah does, however, suggest that pregnant women can make a few changes to their eating habits. 'Although dieting is not appropriate, women can use this special time in their lives to eat more fruit and vegetables and also to cut down on high fat and sugary snacks. They should also take in plenty of dairy products such as milk and yoghurt, but ideally these should be low fat.'

"A slow but sure approach works best"

So how should you go about losing weight if diets are not a good idea? Firstly Sarah explains that people have to set realistic and achievable goals. 'A slow but sure approach works best because weight will then stay off, especially if you increase your level of physical activity.' If you think that this might mean taking out a membership for a fitness club, be reassured. Sarah says 'Very modest amounts of physical activity can make a huge difference to weight loss. Simply parking the car at the far end of the supermarket car park and walking there and back will help.'

Sarah has a three step approach which people find very manageable. 'Any changes however small, that you make will pay off in term of your health. This means that even if you do nothing but eat more fresh fruit and vegetables a day or walk up the stairs instead of taking the lift, you will be making a difference.'

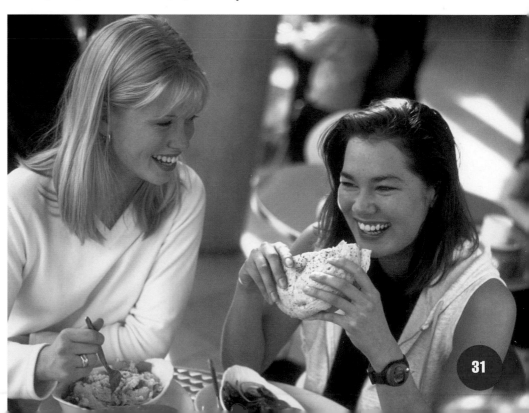

The Three Step Plan

The Three Step Plan is not about dieting, but about making some changes to your eating habits. These will help you to feel good and will make you healthier.

1 Aim not to put on any more weight

Weight creeps up on people. If you can stop putting on any more weight this represents a real achievement. For this first stage, you just need to make some small adjustments to your life. This is not a diet!

- Start to build in more fruit and vegetables into your diet. Think fresh, dried, frozen or tinned fruit, salads and those all-important green vegetables. Eat a fruit, vegetable or salad at every meal.

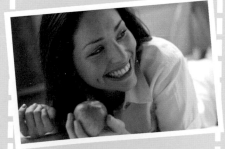

- Switch to semi-skimmed milk or skimmed milk for all or some of the time.
- Try increasing your level of activity just a fraction – walk up those stairs, stop parking in the nearest spot and walk just a little more.

2 Aim to maintain your weight

If you have stopped putting on weight, now try just maintaining your weight. Most women will need around 2,000 calories to maintain their weight, while men will need slightly more, 2,500. Look at our menu below to give you an idea of how much food you will need to eat to maintain your weight.

- Have five portions of fruit and vegetables a day.
- Use skimmed or semi-skimmed milk all the time.
- Make sure that you start the day with breakfast containing slow burning foods such as porridge, banana, breakfast cereals without added sugar.

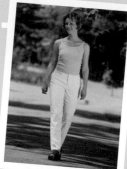

- Eat enough at meal times. Damage is caused by high fat and sugary snacks eaten between meals. If you feel like a snack, have some fresh or dried fruit.
- Get in the habit of walking for half an hour a day. This can be done in three lots of ten minutes rather than all at once. You could also try walking up stairs rather than using the escalator or lift, for example in shops.

A menu for good health

Breakfast (Choose any three from the list)
* Orange juice
* Portion of cereal with semi-skimmed milk
* Slices of toast with scraping of margarine and jam
* Porridge made with semi-skimmed milk
* Poached egg
* Lean grilled bacon

Lunch
* Sandwiches with a low-fat filling such as tuna (avoid mayonnaise, butter or margarine)
Or
* Jacket potato filled with cheese, baked beans or tuna (avoid mayonnaise, butter or margarine)
Or
* Poached egg or baked beans on toast

Followed by
* Low fat yoghurt or low fat dessert
* Fruit

Snacks
* Satsuma, handful of nuts
* Tea cakes or scones with a scraping of butter or dry
* Raisins, apricots,
* Popcorn, unsweetened

Evening meal
* Vegetarian lasagne made with semi-skimmed milk or
* Baked fish or
* Grilled sausages or
* Cottage pie

Served with at least two vegetables such as broccoli, carrots, peas, tomatoes

Small portion of pasta, rice, oven chips, couscous or lentils

* Low fat dessert or yoghurt
* Fresh fruit salad
* Sorbet ice cream
* Greek yoghurt

3 Losing weight

To lose weight, you will need to cut back on your energy or calorie intake. This does not mean that whole groups of food should be cut out or that you will feel hungry. To lose weight, you will probably need foods that add up to around 1,500 calories for women and 1,800 calories for men. This does not mean that you have to count every calorie in everything you eat. In fact calorie counting in this way may leave you feeling very hungry. It's also important not to think that if you have a day where you do eat some high fat, sugary foods, all is lost. Remember that losing weight is very much the 'icing on the cake' and simply by not putting on more weight you are doing very well. It is important not to expect a 'quick fix' and lose weight quickly. The weight you lose gradually is more likely to stay off.

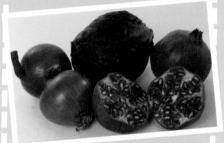

- Use low fat dairy products, such as low fat yoghurt, skimmed or semi-skimmed milk. Make sure you are having at least half a pint (250 mls) of milk a day as well as other dairy foods.
- Make sure that you are eating at least five portions of fresh fruit and vegetables a day. This can be increased by nibbling an apple if you are feeling snackish!
- Make sure that carbohydrate foods such as potatoes, wholemeal bread, rice, pasta, couscous, form the main part of each meal.
- Drink plenty of water and avoid fizzy drinks. Try a slice of lemon in your water.
- Make meal times real events. Sit down and enjoy your food. Avoid eating in front of the television.

Keep an eye on ...

- **Snacks** – these can easily amount to more calories than meals. Have fruit on hand and avoid situations where you eat snacks because you are bored.

- **Alcohol** – wine, beer and other alcoholic drinks are quite high in calories. Once you start to drink, you may also find that you can blow caution to the wind and end up eating fatty foods such as kebabs or a take-away!

- **Fizzy drinks** – even the low calorie versions are not very good for you. Choose water, fruit teas and the odd drink of juice.

Menu @ 1,500 colories for losing weight

Breakfast
* Half a grapefruit
* Unsweetened cereal served with semi-skimmed milk
* Banana

Lunch
* Jacket potato with baked beans
* Green salad, tomatoes and cucumber
* Fruit salad and low fat yoghurt

Evening meal
* Small portion of grilled chicken or fish served with rice, sweet corn and green peppers
* Pasta with a tomato sauce, broccoli and carrots
* Tinned fruit in natural juices and tablespoon of unsweetened, low fat yoghurt

Snacks
* Carrot and celery sticks in low fat yoghurt dip
* Fresh fruit e.g. sliced melon, apple, oranges
* Dried fruits such as raisins, apricots, prunes

Drinks during the day
* Tea, coffee, fruit and herbal teas
* Low fat chocolate drinks
* Fruit juice, sugar-free squashes
* Water, milk
* Fruit smoothies

Keeping up your calcium
You should also have up to one pint (1/2 litre) of semi-skimmed or skimmed milk during the day. This could be taken in tea, coffee or at breakfast with cereal.

LEARNING THE LINGO!

The minute you start reading about balanced diets, a new language appears! Try out our translation service.

CALORIES

This word comes up over and over again. Calories or their official term, Kilocalories (Kcal), are measurements of energy. Foods that are high in calories, for example foods that contain fat, provide the body with lots of energy. You put on weight when you do not use up all the energy that has gone into your body. You lose weight by using more energy that you put into your body. As well as seeing calories on food labels, you may also see the term 'kilojoule'. This is the metric version.

CARBOHYDRATES

Carbohydrate foods are also referred to as starchy foods. They include foods such as bread, cereals, potatoes, rice, pasta, beans and lentils. Carbohydrates give you energy, and fill you up, so it is really important to eat them. Some diets tell you to stop eating carbohydrates, but this is not a good idea at all. Your body will not be getting some important vitamins. Sugar is also a carbohydrate, but because it is so processed, it will give you the energy, but will not fill you up. This is why it is a good idea to limit the amount of sugary foods you eat, especially if they are also high in fat, for example, biscuits, ice cream, chocolate.

FATS

Most people have too much fat in their diet, especially processed and animal fats which are sometimes called saturated fats. This is one reason why people can put on weight, even if they don't eat large amounts of food. A good example of this is crisps. A packet of crisps will probably not fill you up at all, but because it has lots of fat it will give you plenty of calories. Many snack foods, takeaways and processed foods contain a lot of fat, although you may not even realise it. While eating foods that are high in fat can make you put on weight, you should not cut fat out of your diet altogether. Some fat is needed by your body to keep you healthy. It is just a case of getting the balance right. Cut down on animal fats which can cause heart disease, by grilling meat, using semi-skimmed milk and having low fat dairy products. Try also not to add fat when you are cooking or eating. Grill or bake foods rather than frying them. Avoid adding butter, mayonnaise, margarine and high fat salad dressings onto vegetables, bread and salads! People forget that these are fats and so high in calories.

PROTEIN

Protein acts as a body builder and is important. It is found in dairy products, eggs, meat, fish and also beans, pulses, soya, quorn and lentils. If you get your protein from meat and dairy products, it is a good idea to buy lean meats and grill them and switch to low fat dairy products and semi-skimmed milk.

VITAMINS AND MINERALS

Vitamins and minerals are essential for the body. Healthy skin, good teeth and bones and even feeling well is the result of vitamins and minerals. Vitamins and minerals come from a large range of foods, but look out particularly for fresh fruit and vegetables, dairy products and carbohydrates (not sugar). Some vitamins are easily damaged or can escape into the water. To make sure that you are getting your vitamins eat plenty of fresh fruit and, when cooking vegetables, lightly cook them.

Losing weight in order to have a healthy baby may seem a little daunting, but it can be done as Katy Maine tells us.

Katy's story begins in her early twenties when one of her ovaries was removed. 'One night I was in awful pain and was rushed to hospital. They thought that I had appendicitis, but actually it was a cyst on the ovary. Finding out was a terrible shock. I had just woken up and the surgeon came into tell me. My husband came back to find me in floods of tears.' Katy thought that it would be very hard to get pregnant and she got quite depressed. 'I look back now and can see that it was at this point that I began to start eating more. The weight gradually built up, but I didn't really notice it.' Katy's weight soared and she put on an extra three stone (22 kilos). The turning point and motivation for losing weight came out of the blue as Katy explains 'A group of us went for a holiday and I saw a glimpse of myself in my swimming costume in the hotel room. I burst into tears and couldn't face going down to swim. I looked like a Michelin woman and I thought that my friends would think that I was already pregnant.' When Katy got back from holiday, she began to think about losing weight. 'I was determined to do something and so I joined a slimming club. I took a friend for moral support, and they were really friendly and keeping to the diet was easy. I learnt so much about foods and what to eat and what to go carefully on.' Over the next few months Katy gradually lost weight and began to feel better. 'I lost one and then two stone and suddenly everyone was telling me how fantastic I was looking. I was determined to get to my right weight before getting pregnant.' A month after Katy got to her target weight, she became pregnant. ' I was so shocked as I thought it would take forever. I had this new body, was feeling great and then found that I was pregnant. When I went to see my doctor, she said that because I had lost the weight, I would find the pregnancy and birth easier.' Katy watched what she ate during the pregnancy and gave birth to daughter Mia last August. ' I made sure that I ate plenty of fruit and vegetables, gave up alcohol and felt brilliant all through the pregnancy. Knowing that I gave Mia a good start in life makes me feel really proud.'

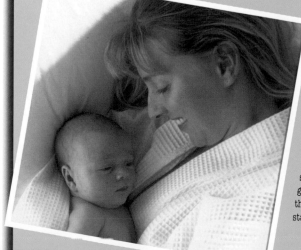

WHAT'S going WRONG?

Cutting down on breakfast is a big mistake.

Ideally, a bowl of unsweetened breakfast cereal served with semi-skimmed milk and some fresh fruit would be a great way to start. Your body needs some slow burning foods. Needing the chocolate bar early on in the day is a big clue that your body is hungry (see also p. 30).

YOUR ATTITUDES TOWARDS FOOD ARE PART OF YOUR PROBLEM.

Having the occasional slice of cream cake is fine. Taking the other because you don't like waste is not so healthy. There is not a nationwide shortage of food and cream cakes are likely to be around for a long time to come! You also started the day believing that you had to restrict yourself. This is the main reason why diets fail. This was not realistic and so has probably made you far too aware of foods. This accounts for the biscuit eating in the afternoon. You might also have been bored which can be deadly!

TIP Identify times when you are eating because you are bored. Think about an alternative to food in these times.

You may also need to become aware of money and food. Choosing something that is high fat or sugary just because it is on special offer should be avoided. Being overweight could be far more costly for you and your baby (see also p. 30 about attitudes towards food).

LUNCH IS HIGH IN FATS AND LOW IN FRESH FRUIT AND VEGETABLES.

Whilst meat can be good for you, the pastry is very high in fat. A sandwich containing meat and salad would have been a better option or a jacket potato with a low fat filling such as tuna or baked beans. The low fat crisps might seem a good bet, but they do not fill you up and still contain plenty of fat. The strawberry cheesecake is both high in fat and sugar. Whilst if you had really fancied it, you could have had it, but remember that you have already had a cream cake. Fresh fruit or a low-fat yoghurt would have been a much better idea. Water would have been much more helpful for your body to digest food as well as being good for your skin. Tap water is also free!

TIP Remember that you do not have to end a meal with something sweet. See if you can break this as a habit. Try instead to have more of the main course.

TEA WAS EATEN ON THE HOOF!

The trouble with eating on the way home, in front of the television or doing something else means that you are not concentrating on the food. This means that later on you can feel as if you have not had a lot to eat. This is why you probably wanted something else to eat. Take time out to sit and enjoy meal times.

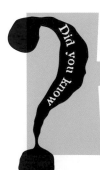

Did you know

Skimmed milk has half the calories of whole milk, but more calcium, an essential mineral for strong bones and teeth.

The average chocolate bar can be the equivalent in calories of half a meal!

One glass of fruit juice is the equivalent to one orange.

There is no difference in the number of calories between margarine or butter.

Children perform better at school if they have eaten breakfast?

Having one pint (half a litre) of milk a day will help prevent osteoporosis (brittle bones) in later life?

Fat contains more than twice as many calories as sugar?

THERE'S A DIET ABOUT

Look in any magazine or bookshop and you will find that a new diet is being advertised. But do they work and are they safe?

We look at four different methods of dieting and ask our expert, Sarah Fulton, for her opinion.

Want to lose weight quickly?
Phone 0785 000009987

Slimming replacement meals

These are drinks that you take instead of having a meal. They claim rapid weight loss.

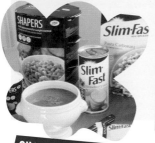

Our expert says

This is a short-term measure that invariably results in weight being put on quickly afterwards. Users often feel that they have failed after using this type of product because they cannot sustain such a restrictive diet and because the later weight gain is more than the weight that is lost. The danger with these products is that no attempt is made to address the real issues as to why weight has gone on in the first place.

Score 0/10

Slimming books

Slimming books offer guidance and recipes to help weight loss.

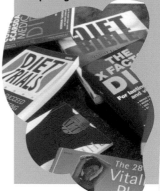

Our expert says

Advice in slimming books can vary enormously. Some books can be very motivational and helpful, although people should choose with care.
Avoid books which promise quick weight loss or ones which cut out groups of foods. Fad diet books come and go, so be very cautious when looking at them. Choose books that promote healthy eating and advise slow but gradual weight loss. Remember too that diets that are very restrictive will not be sustainable and so may encourage binge eating.

Score ?/10 Impossible to give as it depends on the quality of advice given.

Slimming pills

Pills that claim to help you lose weight.

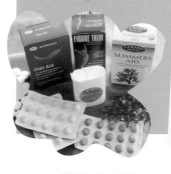

Our expert says

Slimming pills that are advertised in magazines and newspapers are potentially dangerous as well as expensive. Their exaggerated claims often have no scientific basis and even pills that claim to be 'natural' can cause reactions and so should be avoided, especially for anyone hoping to become pregnant. Anyone taking such pills should tell their doctor in case they react with any existing medication.

Slimming clubs

Slimming clubs work by providing advice and guidance to members.

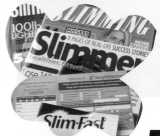

Our expert says

Reputable slimming clubs can really make a difference to some people. They provide an incentive to lose weight while also being good social occasions. It is important to choose a good slimming club. Avoid any clubs that promise very quick weight loss or ones where whole food groups are excluded from the diet.

Score 9/10

Our expert's conclusion

Many products such as slimming pills and rapid weight loss programmes look too good to be true. This is because they are. The only safe way to lose weight is to get the balance right between the amount of food you eat and the amount of energy that you are using. Promises of quick weight loss will result in water being lost from the body rather than actual fat. Rapid weight loss is nearly always followed by rapid weight gain and so can leave people being heavier than they were at the start.

Slimming clubs and slimming books that encourage slower weight loss are therefore winners. Gradual and sensible weight loss should mean that people can still enjoy their food and not find themselves 'yo-yo' dieting.

FAT FACTS

Most people can only safely lose 2lb (1kg) of fat in a week.

Contrary to popular belief, it is easier for the body to lose weight than to gain it!

Fast tips

TO A HEALTHY YOU!

1 Include low fat dairy products in your diet

These are essential for strengthening your bones and teeth, and for helping your baby to develop. Choose low fat products as these have fewer calories.

2 Aim to have five different portions of fruit and vegetables a day

Fruit and vegetables are amazingly good for vitamins and minerals. Wash them carefully and avoid overcooking vegetables.

3 Don't eat in front of the television

Make sure that your body and mind know when you are eating. Eating while doing something else means that you will not notice that you have eaten and may end up feeling hungry.

4 Build up your activity level

Every single extra step that you take will help you on the road to fitness and also to losing weight. Walk just a little further than usual or try going up the stairs. Build up the exercise until you are walking about half an hour a day, even if you do it in three batches of ten minutes.

5 Eat carbohydrates such as bread, rice, potatoes and pasta at each meal

Foods containing unprocessed carbohydrates such as bread, pasta, lentils and rice are fantastic. They fill you up, provide slow-release energy and give you much-needed vitamins! Make sure that they form the basis of any meal, for example, a jacket potato with baked beans or a sandwich with tuna and salad.

6 Eat regularly, don't skip meals

Skipping meals will mean that you are likely to snack. Because you are so hungry, you are likely to choose snacks that are high in fat and sugar.

7 Avoid alcohol

Alcohol contains nearly as many calories as fat. It also weakens good intentions. Remember too, that alcohol can reduce your ability to conceive and may also damage the baby in the early stages of pregnancy.

8 Keep an eye on snacks

Snacks often add up over a day to more calories than the meals that you have eaten. Watch out for chocolate bars, crisps and breakfast bars. If you have had some of these snacks, increase your activity level, but don't cut back on meals.

Fact or fiction

There are many myths about losing weight. Try our quick quiz.

1 You should avoid dairy products if you want to lose weight. 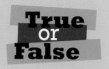 *True or False*

2 You should always eat a good breakfast. *True or False*

3 Lower fat crisps are good for you. 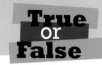 *True or False*

4 An average meal comes to about 350-400 calories. 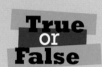 *True or False*

5 Eating bread and pasta will make you fat. 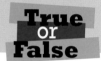 *True or False*

Answers

1 FALSE Dairy products are essential and should not be cut out. Switch to low fat options.

2 TRUE Starting the day with breakfast will stop you from snacking later on. Breakfast should contain slow-burning carbohydrates such as muesli, porridge and sugar-free breakfast cereals. You should also have some semi-skimmed or skimmed milk and some fruit for a great start.

3 FALSE Lower fat crisps, biscuits and even ready-made meals often contain a lot of fat although it may be less than the standard ones. Choose fresh fruit for snacks wherever possible.

4 TRUE Most people's meals are about 350-450 calories. When people put on weight the problem is due to snacking in between meals or that the meals contain too much hidden fat (for example, the odd knob of butter added to vegetables).

5 FALSE Breads, pasta and potatoes will not make you fat unless you eat huge quantities of them. It is what goes with them, such as the mayonnaise or creamy sauces, that may be fattening. They will fill you up and so prevent you from snacking.

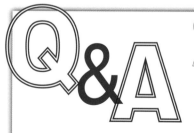

Q Help! I have just found out that I am pregnant and I am four stone overweight.

A Don't worry and certainly do not go and start a restrictive diet. Use the next few months to change your lifestyle and eating habits though. Use this as an opportunity not only to have a new baby, but also to have a new you!

If you have not started taking folic acid supplements, begin now until you are twelve weeks pregnant. Next, begin to walk a little more and take small steps towards getting fit. Every step you take towards being more active will pay huge dividends. You can also adjust what you eat slightly. Buy semi-skimmed milk as this has more calcium in it, and get at least five portions of fruit and vegetables onto your plate each day. Cut out high fat snacks and alcohol from your diet. Your baby needs real food, full of vitamins and minerals not empty calories.

Q I am underweight. My friends tell me that I can put on weight by eating more chocolate.

A Contrary to popular belief, being underweight can be a problem. It can be harder to conceive as some women may have irregular periods if they are very underweight. Putting on weight means taking in more calories. While you can put on weight by eating high fat snack foods such as chocolate, this is not a good idea for several reasons, not least of all the health of your teeth. First, if you eat chocolate you will not get important nutrients such as vitamin C, folic acid and iron. Secondly, once you are at your optimum weight, you may have got into the habit of eating it.

For the moment, try adding more calories into your your diet by using whole fat milk and dairy products, and by looking for foods which contain high levels of natural oils such as olives, avocados and nuts. Try cooking with olive oil or other vegetable oils and eating more oily fish. Remember though, that once you have reached your ideal weight, you will then need to switch back to low fat foods. It might also be a good idea to consult your doctor if you are very underweight so that he/she can give you a health check as well as advice.

Foods for a flying start

The old saying 'you are what you eat' really has some meaning when it comes to conception and pregnancy. There is plenty of research to show that the foods that you eat before and during pregnancy can influence the health of a baby. We look at the ways in which you can help your baby to get off to a flying start.

Deficiencies can have serious knock on effects
It is now known that the body needs a vast array of chemicals in order to remain in tip-top health. The chemicals themselves can be grouped into five types: vitamins, minerals, proteins, fats and carbohydrates.
In some cases the quantities required of particular vitamins and minerals are quite small, but an absence or deficiency can have some serious knock on effects. A good example of this is zinc. Men who do not have sufficient zinc in their diets can have low sperm counts, while a lack of folic acid in a woman's diet can affect the developing baby or fetus.

SURPLUS TO REQUIREMENTS

While deficiencies of particular chemicals can cause the body problems, so too can a surplus. A good example of this is fat. If we take in too many fatty and sugary foods, the body ends up having to store them as fat. It is known that an excess of fat can lower your chances of conception and of having a healthy pregnancy. Some chemicals, such as vitamin A, can also be poisonous if taken in very high dosages. This is why eating products which contain animal livers is no longer recommended for pregnant women.

MEALS PROVIDE A CHEMICAL PACKAGE

Some of the chemicals that the body takes in from food work alongside each other in order to be effective. A good example of this is iron. Most people know that iron is really important for women, but many do not know that it is absorbed more easily when it is taken with foods containing vitamin C such as fruit and vegetables. Luckily, by eating healthy meals with plenty of fruit and vegetables you can automatically give the body what it needs. Because meals provide you with a complex chemical package, you should avoid going on diets which work by eating a limited number of foods. In the same way, an ultra low fat diet is not recommended as many vitamins are absorbed with fat.

ALCOHOL INTERFERES WITH THE ABSORPTION OF VITAMINS

While some chemicals work together, others do not. Alcohol, for example, can interfere with the work of vitamins. This is why couples who are planning to conceive are advised to cut down or avoid it.

FRESH IS BEST

Finally, it is also worth knowing that the way that food is prepared can make a difference to what is in it. Packaged and canned foods, while appearing to be quick and easy, do not have the same levels of vitamins and minerals as freshly-cooked food. They often contain high levels of fat, salt and sugar. So 'fresh is best' is a key message. This may mean spending a little longer in the kitchen, but may be you could try to cooking with your partner. Preparing food together is a great way of building relationships.

SO HOW DO YOU ACHIEVE A BALANCED DIET?

Fortunately, you do not need to be a scientist to make sure that your diet is balanced. Foods can be divided into groups and you need to take foods from across each group.

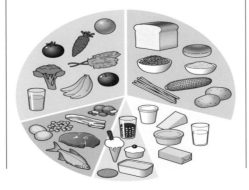

VEGETARIANS AND VEGANS

If you are a vegetarian or a vegan, it will be important to seek nutritional advice before and after conception. This is because you are likely to need supplements to ensure that you are getting enough of some key vitamins, especially vitamin B12, iron and zinc. Vitamin B12 can be a particular problem because it is commonly found in animal products such as meat and eggs, although some can be found in yeast. A lack of vitamin B12 can cause fetal abnormalities so it is really worth taking some advice about how best to incorporate it into your diet.

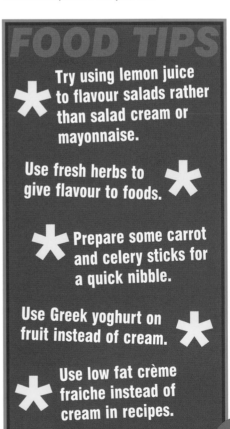

FOOD TIPS

* Try using lemon juice to flavour salads rather than salad cream or mayonnaise.

* Use fresh herbs to give flavour to foods.

* Prepare some carrot and celery sticks for a quick nibble.

* Use Greek yoghurt on fruit instead of cream.

* Use low fat crème fraiche instead of cream in recipes.

diet and conception

There are ways that you and your partner can maximise your chances of conception by looking at your diet. First of all you should check that you are eating a balanced diet and are both at a healthy weight.

Look out too for the following:

Alcohol ✗
- Can seriously reduce chances of conception as it damages some essential vitamins
- May damage fetus

Avoid or cut down

Foods high in refined sugar ✗
- Can decrease chances of conception
- Can affect development of unborn baby
- Can prevent vitamins and minerals from being taken in

Avoid or cut down

Caffeine products such as coffee ✗
- Can reduce conception
- Linked to early miscarriages

Avoid or cut down

Folic acid ✓
- Helps healthy development of fetus
- Cuts the risk of the unborn baby developing spina bifida (neural tube defects)

Women should take 0.4mg supplements before conceiving and also during early pregnancy.
Eat plenty of green vegetables.

Zinc ✓
- May improve male fertility
- Helps healthy development of fetus

Zinc is found in wholegrain bread, meat, cheese, eggs and milk

Oily fish ✓
- Links to male fertility
- Helps healthy development of fetus

Eat at least 300g of oily fish such as sardines, mackerel, salmon and herring a week

WATCH OUT FOODS TO AVOID EATING

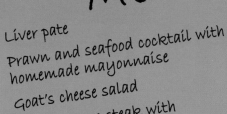

MENU

Liver pate
Prawn and seafood cocktail with homemade mayonnaise
Goat's cheese salad
Medium rare steak with green salad
Ploughman's lunch with brie, stilton and camembert cheese
Homemade chocolate mousse

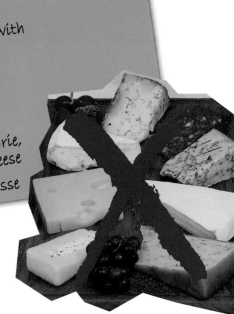

It's lunchtime and the local café is busy. Although you are very hungry, let's look at the menu first. Some dishes may not be good for you if you are trying to get pregnant or are already pregnant.

It may seem surprising, but some foods are not advised during pregnancy or for women who are likely to be so, even though they can safely be eaten at other times. This is because they may harbour bacteria or contain substances that are not desirable. So which foods should women avoid and why?

Foods associated with food poisoning

Some foods are particularly associated with food poisoning. This is because some raw foods can have high levels of dangerous bacteria such as Salmonella, E. coli and Campylobacter. These bacteria can cause serious infections with sickness and diarrhoea being the most common symptoms. Unfortunately, these infections can also cause miscarriages or stillbirths.

- Undercooked eggs. For example, fried eggs with runny yolks, soft boiled eggs, home-made mayonnaise, desserts made with raw eggs such as chocolate mousse or tiramisu.
- Undercooked meat. For example rare or medium rare steak. Watch out particularly for chicken and turkey and check that they are piping hot and cooked all the way through.
- Barbecued meats unless you are really sure that they are cooked all the way through.
- Unpasteurised milk and cheese products.
- Shellfish such as mussels and prawns, even if they are cooked.

Foods associated with listeria

Listeria is another bacteria, which again can be harmful to the unborn child. While food poisoning usually gives people sickness and diarrhoea, listeria gives people flu-like symptoms. The infection can cause miscarriage and stillbirth in pregnant women, although fortunately this is reasonably rare.

- Ripened soft cheeses such as Brie, Camembert, Stilton, Danish Blue.
- Unpasteurised milk and cheeses.
- Pre-packed salads unless you wash them again.

Foods linked to toxoplasmosis

Toxoplasmosis is an organism that can be found in the soil, but also in raw meat and unpasteurised milk. It causes a flu-like infection that as well as causing miscarriage can also cause damage to the developing baby.

- Unwashed fruit and vegetables.
- Undercooked meat (see box on left).
- Unpasteurised milk.

As well as foods that may cause infections, there are also a few foods that are not recommended as they may affect the baby.

- Liver and liver products such as pate.
- Liver should be avoided as it contains high levels of vitamin A.

? Peanuts and products such as peanut butter.

Some children are born with an allergy to peanuts. This is quite a serious allergy as it can affect breathing. It is thought that by avoiding peanuts and peanut products, you can reduce the risk of your child developing this allergy.

? Coffee.

While the odd cup of coffee should not be a problem, drinking more than three cups of strong coffee a day should be avoided. It is thought that high levels of caffeine may be linked to early miscarriage and even to Sudden Infant Death Syndrome.

The threat in your kitchen

It would be easy to imagine that food poisoning outbreaks affect restaurants, hospitals and other outside catering spots. But this is not the case. We are most likely to get food poisoning in our own homes. We ask Arthur Atkins, Principal Environmental Health Officer for some advice.

According to Arthur Atkins, some very simple measures can prevent food poisoning. 'Cross contamination is a major reason why people get food poisoning. Bacteria are literally moved from one food source to another without anyone realising it. Take people's hands. If they have touched raw meat and then begin washing a salad, the salad will now have bacteria on it from the meat.' Arthur suggests that you should wash your hands at the start of any food preparation and after touching raw items. He also reminds people about working surfaces and tools, 'A knife and chopping board might be used to cut up some raw poultry and many people will go onto chop up other things on the same board. Any bacteria will be moved onto the next food.'

As well as thinking about food preparation, Arthur also suggests that people need to think about their fridges. 'The golden rule is to keep raw things away from cooked items. Raw meat should be covered and stored on the bottom shelf, while things that will be eaten without being cooked need to go above. Unfortunately, many fridges are designed with the salad drawer at the very bottom. This can mean that blood from uncovered meat can drip onto salad items. It is best to cover up meat and think about putting salad higher up.'

When it comes to checking that meat and poultry are properly cooked, Arthur suggests investing in a meat thermometer. 'One easy step to take is to buy a simple meat thermometer from a kitchen shop or supermarket. Checking that meat and other dishes are cooked to at least 75-80°C will ensure that bacteria will be killed off. Too often, people think that things are cooked when they are not really.' He also says that recent tests done on poultry means that the standard advice about looking to see if juices run clear may not be accurate enough. 'Before it was thought that if juices from meat ran clear, the meat would be thoroughly cooked. This is not the case though and so again, the best way is to check with a thermometer.'

As well as looking at the danger of undercooked meat, Arthur also warns about the dangers of fruit and vegetables, 'People think that because they are not meat, that they don't really have to be washed. In fact because salads and fruit are not cooked, any bacteria or organisms will not be killed off. Some salads and tomatoes are imported with quite high levels of potentially dangerous bacteria.'

Finally, Arthur is not a fan of barbecues. 'There is a real danger that whilst meat may be cooked on the outside, it is not properly cooked inside. This means that bacteria have not been killed.'

FOOD HANDLING TIPS

- Always wash your hands before preparing and serving food.
- Wash your hands, knives and chopping boards immediately after preparing raw meat.
- Keep any cuts on hands covered using plasters.
- Cook meat thoroughly and check using a meat thermometer, 80°C will be safe.
- Store raw foods and cooked foods separately.

Just how good is your food handling?

Test yourself in our fun quiz.

1 You've decided to make a salad. Do you:

a) wash each leaf carefully making sure there is no soil or dirt

b) buy a ready prepared one from the supermarket and put it straight into the bowl

c) stick the whole thing under the tap and give it a quick shake?

2 You are out shopping for food. Do you:

a) check the best before dates, look carefully at labels and think about healthy food

b) wander around looking for bargains, although sometimes you end up throwing out food

c) buy only reduced for quick sale items as it doesn't really matter about the dates?

3 You have just come in from doing the shopping. Do you:

a) sort out the food carefully e.g. put raw meat on separate shelf in fridge

b) open the fridge door and just try to cram things in wherever there is a space

c) leave the shopping for a few hours until you have had a chance to make a cup of tea and had a chat on the phone?

4 You drop a piece of cooked fish onto the floor. Do you:

a) throw it out and think of something else to eat

b) give it a quick wash, put it on the plate and hope no one will notice

c) pop it back onto the plate as it will have more flavour now?

5 You have just finished chopping up some meat. Do you:

a) wash your hands, the chopping board and the knife you used

b) get out another chopping board and wipe your hands on your apron

c) cut up a few more vegetables whilst the chopping board and knife are out?

6 There is just one portion of a reheated meal left in the dish. Do you:

a) throw it out because it has now been cooked twice

b) put it in the fridge, but thoroughly cook it the next day

c) leave it out and have it in a few days time?

7 You notice hairs on a cream cake that you bought earlier. Do you:

a) feel disgusted and take the cake back to the shop and complain

b) only eat the bottom part of the cake where there were no hairs

c) pull off the hairs and enjoy the cake? After all they could have been yours.

SO HOW DID YOU DO?

Mostly As

Wow, we'd definitely like to come round to you for dinner. You have a good understanding of how to prepare and cook food safely. All this will come in very handy as when babies are being weaned, it is essential that they are given safe food.

Mostly Bs

You've got some idea, but you really need to think food safety before trying to save money. Make sure that you are heating food to high enough temperatures. Remember too that raw meat and poultry and anything that they have touched can contaminate other foods. This means that chopping boards, plates and knives need to be washed once they have been used for raw meat, poultry and fish. As a lot of contamination is is spread on the hands, think about washing your hands when you have touched raw meat etc. Simply wiping hands is not good enough.

Mostly Cs

You need to keep a good stock of toilet paper in your home as diarrhoea might strike at any time. Seriously though, food poisoning is actually very dangerous and could cost you the life of your unborn child. It's actually quite easy to get into good food hygiene routines and you will know that your food is really safe. Read our article on p. 44 to get more tips.

Eating out SAFELY

PREPARING YOUR OWN FOOD AT HOME IS THE BEST WAY OF KNOWING THAT THE FOOD YOU EAT IS SAFE. BUT WHAT SHOULD YOU DO IF YOU WANT TO EAT OUT? HERE ARE SOME OF ARTHUR'S TIPS.

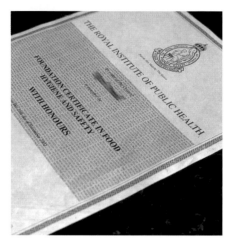

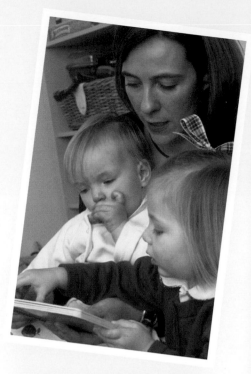

Jane 28 has two daughters, Betsy 3 and Katie 15 months

'It was a warm sunny day and I was just three months pregnant with our second daughter. We had decided to go to the park and have a picnic. I thought it would be nice to buy some cakes on the way as a treat. I had only just stopped getting morning sickness. I popped into the baker's and saw the cream cakes in the window. Looking back now, I can still see them in my mind's eye. They were in the sun, but of course I didn't think about that.

I bought one for me and doughnuts for everyone else. Later at about four o'clock, I began to feel sick. Then, about half an hour later, I began to be sick. I was violently sick, on and on until there was nothing to bring up. I couldn't keep water down and after about three hours of non-stop vomiting I noticed that I was starting to spot blood. I phoned the emergency doctor who came out straight away. He decided to give me a sedative to stop the vomiting as he thought that otherwise I might have a miscarriage. I was really scared that I would lose the baby. Fortunately, the injection worked quite quickly and everything was fine, although I started to be really careful about what I ate when I was out. It was scary to think that one cream cake could have cost me my baby.'

FOOD HYGIENE AWARDS

Look out for Food hygiene award certificates on the walls. This shows that some of the staff have had training in food hygiene. In some parts of the country this is compulsory.

HEARTBEAT AWARDS

Heartbeat awards are given to restaurants who can offer a no-smoking area, a menu approved by a nutritionist and have shown that they have a high standard of food handling.

CLEANLINESS AND TIDINESS

Look at how tidy and clean any eating area is. If what you can see is dirty and poor, imagine what it might be like behind closed doors!

FOOD ON DISPLAY

Look to see how food is being displayed. If you are concerned, ask about when items were made or how long they have been out. It is usually best to be patient and have something cooked on the spot, rather than eat something that has been warming for a while.

Avoid getting traveller's tummy!

Relaxing abroad may be one way to enjoy conceiving a baby, but make sure that you do not get food poisoning.

As well as checking that restaurants and fast food places are clean, you can also help yourself by taking these simple precautions:

Avoid salads and fruit unless you know that they have been properly washed

Drink bottled water and avoid ice cubes

Avoid soft ice creams

Ask for meat to be well cooked

Avoid shellfish, especially mussels and oysters.

FOOD MATTERS

We answer your food questions

Q I am worried because I got quite drunk when I didn't know that I was pregnant. Will this have harmed the baby?

A In an ideal world, women are told to avoid alcohol if they are hoping to conceive and also during pregnancy. This is because repeated exposure to high levels of alcohol has been known to cause fetal abnormalities. The chances are that your baby will be fine, but you should avoid any further alcohol during the pregnancy. If you are still concerned about your pregnancy, talk to your doctor or midwife.

Q I have always been on and off diets. Now I am pregnant and want to diet again. Can you recommend a safe diet for me?

A Even if you are overweight, the advice is to avoid going on a diet. Try instead to improve the quality of what you eat. Look out for fresh fruit and vegetables and cut back on high fat and sugary snacks. Eat proper meals and do not binge or use laxatives. You should also seek some further advice because repeated dieting may have left your body lacking in vitamins such as B12 or minerals such as calcium. Do this as a priority so that you can give your baby a flying start. We suggest you also think about getting some professional help about your feelings towards food and your body. This is important because caring for a baby is physically and emotionally demanding and you owe it to yourself and your baby to feel good about yourself.

Q I think I am several weeks pregnant. Is it too late to take folic acid?

A No, start straight away! Folic acid has many benefits in pregnancy. This is why women are encouraged to take 400mcg a day before they become pregnant and during the first weeks of pregnancy.

Q I have heard that being on the pill can lower your levels of vitamin B12. Is this true?

A Yes, women who have just stopped taking the pill (oral contraceptive) can be lacking in B12. This means that if you have come off the pill to get pregnant, you should make sure that your diet contains eggs, meat and oily fish. Seek further advice if you are a vegetarian or vegan as the chances are you will need to take a supplement.

Q I am a vegetarian. How can I make sure that I have everything in my diet?

A Everyone needs a balanced diet, whether or not they are pregnant or hoping to conceive. Vegetarians and vegans often need to check that their diet contains enough vitamin B12, iron, protein and calcium. Consider asking your doctor for advice about balancing your diet as it is crucial to your baby's development that you are taking in enough nutrients.

Q I am confused about which fats are safe and how much fat I should be having in my diet.

A The reason why you may be confused is that some fats are better for us than others. Fats found in animal products such as milk, eggs, cheese and meat are called saturated fats. These fats are known to contribute to heart disease, obesity and cancer. You can cut down on these fats by choosing low fat yoghurts, semi-skimmed milk, choosing lean meats and grilling rather than frying. The type of fats that should be in your diet should come from plants and oily fish.

Q Should I be taking a multi-vitamin supplement?

A It is not really necessary if you are otherwise eating well. A balanced diet containing at least five portions of fruit and vegetables should give you everything you need. Taking multi-vitamins will not harm you providing you take only the recommended dose.

Q My friend is on a 'no fat' diet and is losing lots of weight. I've heard that this can be bad for you – is this true? What should I suggest to her?

A While your friend may lose some weight now, she is likely to put it back on over the next few months. Having no fat also means that she is likely to be lacking in some key vitamins. Encourage her to try our Three Step Plan (see page 32) and lose weight more naturally. This way, the weight she loses may stay off.

The FOLIC ACID Story

Daily folic acid supplements are an absolute must for women who are hoping to conceive or who are already pregnant. We look at the exciting story behind this piece of crucial advice.

It's breakfast time. Anna takes a sip of orange juice and pops a 400mcg tablet of folic acid into her mouth. She's been doing this everyday since deciding to start a family. Yesterday her first scan showed that the baby is absolutely fine.

Anna's unborn baby is benefiting from a medical breakthrough: the discovery that folic acid is needed for the healthy development of a fetus.

For many years, doctors had been puzzled as to why some babies were born with neural tube defects, such as spina bifida, to apparently healthy women of all ages. Neural tube defects affect the ability of the brain to pass information down through the spine. In extreme cases, babies cannot survive after they are born, while in less severe cases babies may have some paralysis.

Today, it is known that folic acid is absolutely crucial in early pregnancy to help the neural tube to close and the spine of the unborn child to form properly. As this happens between the 25th and 30th day after conception, many women will not even know that they are pregnant. This is why all women are urged to take daily folic acid supplements when they are planning to get pregnant.

The folic acid story continues. Researchers are finding that there are some indications that folic acid may also reduce the risk of other birth defects, such as cleft lip and palate, and certain heart defects. Folic acid may also play a role in protecting against some forms of cancer and heart disease.

So is the folic acid story near its end? Not at all! While the numbers of babies being born with spina bifida and other neural tube defects has fallen considerably, the message still needs to be broadcast. So if you know someone who is thinking about getting pregnant, get them to pick up some folic acid tablets from the chemist.

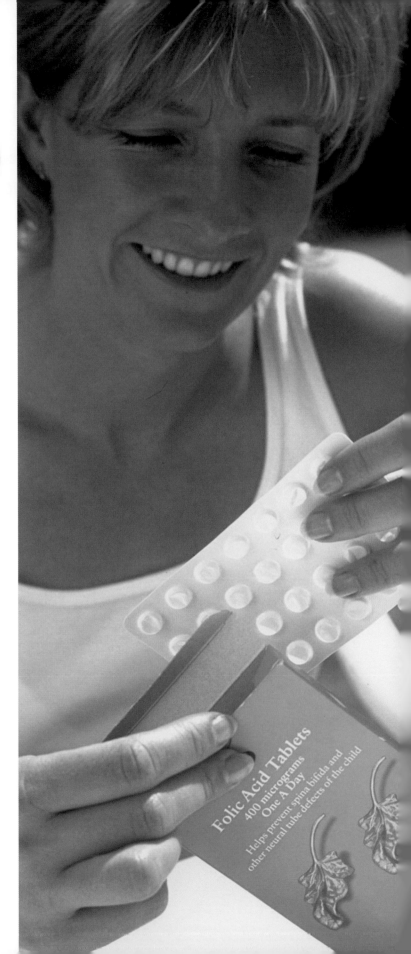

Folic Acid Tablets
400 micrograms
One A Day
Helps prevent spina bifida and other neural tube defects of the child

Folic acid fact file

What is folic acid?
Folic acid, sometimes referred to as folate, is an essential vitamin B. It is essential for the healthy development of the fetus.

How much folic acid should I take?
400 micrograms a day, taken in one tablet.

Where can I get it?
From your local chemist or ask your doctor.

What will it do?
It will reduce by as much as 70% the chances of having a baby with spina bifida, cleft palate and hare lip. It may also help your heart and help you to beat off cancer.

When should it be taken?
Ideally, it should be taken before you get pregnant. But if you are already pregnant, you should still take it up to the twelfth week of pregnancy.

Are there any side effects?
No. Your body will get rid of any excess.

Is it possible to get it naturally?
Yes, providing your diet is high in the foods listed below and that the foods are eaten raw or very lightly cooked. Taking a supplement acts as a good insurance policy and so is recommended.

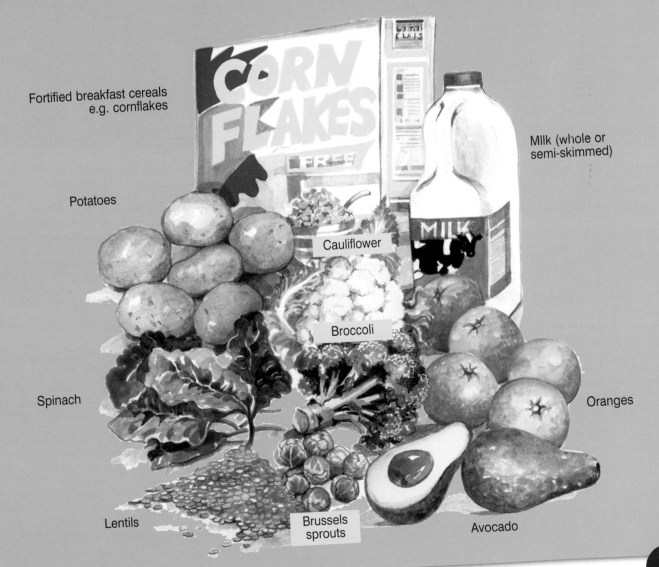

Fortified breakfast cereals e.g. cornflakes

Milk (whole or semi-skimmed)

Potatoes

Cauliflower

Broccoli

Spinach

Oranges

Lentils

Brussels sprouts

Avocado

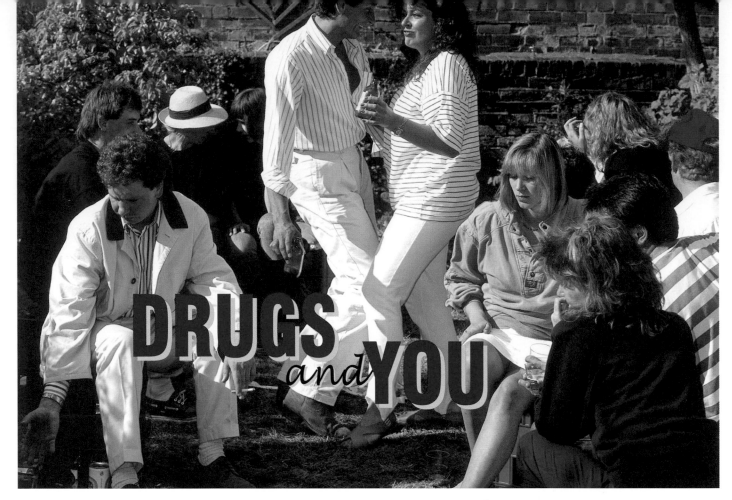

DRUGS and YOU

Drugs are almost part of our everyday life. Paracetamol and aspirin can be found in the petrol station while coffee shops are everywhere. But if you are thinking about getting pregnant or are in early pregnancy, now is the time to think about what you are putting in to your body.

FERTILITY CAN BE AFFECTED BY DRUGS

Most people can see the sense in stopping smoking and taking drugs during pregnancy, but surprisingly, some substances such as alcohol and tobacco can actually make conceiving a baby a whole lot harder. If you are trying for a baby, it is also important to watch out what you are taking , because for a period of at least two weeks, you will not know that you are pregnant. This is because there is a time lapse of two weeks between conception and missing your period.

THE FIRST WEEKS

During pregnancy, everything that is taken into the mother's body can be passed on to the growing embryo. This is why having a healthy diet is important as the embryo requires good nutrition.

It also means that chemicals contained in things such as alcohol, aspirin and herbal products can affect the embryo, even in quite small quantities. The first twelve weeks are an especially important time in an embryo's life as essential organs and structures are being formed in this time.

So what should you look out for:

COFFEE AND CAFFEINE PRODUCTS

Coffee, energy drinks and some soft drinks can contain high levels of the stimulant caffeine. There is some research to show that taking in caffeine can lower your chances of conceiving. It is also thought that high levels of caffeine may be in some way responsible for some miscarriages. While two or three cups a day are fine, you may want to avoid drinking more than that.

OVER THE COUNTER DRUGS

Medicines such as paracetamol have been licensed for over the counter use. They are generally harmless, but it is wise to check the labels and also to ask for some advice, particularly in the first twelve weeks of a pregnancy. If you are not sure, ask your chemist if they are safe in early pregnancy or make an appointment to see your doctor if you feel you need to take medication. Remember that doctors are not mind readers so that unless you tell them that you are trying for a baby, they will not necessarily prescribe medication that is safe in early pregnancy!

MEDICATION PRESCRIBED BY THE DOCTOR

You may be taking medication that has been prescribed by your doctor. If you know that you are likely to get pregnant or if you have done a test and know that you are pregnant, you should make an urgent appointment to see your doctor. It is not a good idea to suddenly stop taking medication especially if you have a condition such as epilepsy, diabetes, high blood pressure or asthma. Your doctor will check whether the prescribed medication is suitable for pregnant women and if not will change it.

ALCOHOL

If you are a heavy or even moderate drinker now is the time to cut down or even better stop drinking altogether. Cutting back on alcohol can positively improve your chances of getting pregnant. Secondly heavy drinking and binge drinking, especially in those first twelve weeks, can be a factor in miscarriages and may damage the developing embryo.

HERBAL MEDICINES AND TEAS

While fruit teas are fine, go carefully on herbal products and medicines. Double-check whether or not they are suitable in early pregnancy. It's easy to forget that herbs in the wrong combination can be poisonous even if they are made out of natural products. They are, after all, used in making many of today's modern drugs. If you are unsure, either steer clear or ask a qualified herbalist or your family doctor.

TOBACCO

Put simply, you need to give up or cut down on smoking. Smoking cigarettes and other tobacco products affects men's fertility and so chances of conception can be reduced. In early pregnancy, you run the risk of miscarriage, while later on in pregnancy you may give birth prematurely or have a low birth weight baby. Later on, some babies that appear healthy at birth can die, apparently for no reason, in cot deaths. If you want to think about giving up, have a look on p.63 for some tips.

STREET DRUGS

Street drugs are of course illegal, and their effects on the unborn baby can be very harmful. Remember that anything that you are taking when pregnant can get through to the developing baby. In the case of some categories of drugs, such as heroin, they can interfere with the ability to conceive in the first place. Other drugs, such as cannabis, which some people feel are reasonably safe, may not be when you are pregnant or trying to conceive. Cannabis especially when taken with tobacco may increase your risk of miscarriage.

Although some people think ecstasy is a mild drug, it should also be avoided. Ecstasy along with other drugs that stimulate the body's senses and give you boundless energy can mean that your body is not resting enough and you may not feel like eating. This has knock-on effects for the developing embryo which needs plenty of regular nutrition.

If you or your partner do take drugs on a regular basis, now could be a good time to think about changing your lifestyle. Caring for a baby is not only tiring, but quite expensive and drugs are not cheap. The good news is that drugs agencies and health professionals such as doctors and midwives are keen to help women and their partners when they are pregnant or thinking about starting a family. If stopping or cutting down on drugs is likely to be difficult, consider getting some help. A good starting point is to begin by calling the National Drugs Helpline. Their latest helpline 'Frank' is a free phone number 0800 77 66 00. Alternatively visit their website on www.talktofrank.com

Quick guide

Avoiding drugs which may be harmful is essential in the first twelve weeks in a pregnancy. Our guide gives some general advice, but if you are unsure as to what to do, consult your doctor. Do not stop taking prescribed drugs. Always visit your doctor first.

Drug	What you should do?
Amphetamines (speed, whiz)	Avoid and stop using.
Anti-convulsants (for epilepsy)	Do not stop taking, but visit doctor immediately.
Aspirin	Best avoided or check with doctor.
Cocaine (coke)	Avoid and stop using.
Coffee and drinks containing caffeine e.g. energy drinks	2-3 cups of coffee a day. Cut down on caffeine drinks.
Cold and flu relief products	Check with chemist or doctor before taking.
Ecstasy	Avoid and stop using.
Herbal medicines, teas	Read labels carefully. Check with doctor.
Ibuprofen/Nurofen	Check with chemist or doctor.
Laxatives, diet tablets	Avoid and stop using.
Methadone and heroin	Visit doctor immediately.
Paracetamol	Check with chemist or doctor.
Steroids (including inhalers for asthma)	Do not stop taking, but visit doctor immediately.
Tobacco	Stop or cut down.
Tranquilisers (Valium, Prozac)	Do not stop taking, but visit doctor immediately.

Drinking up time

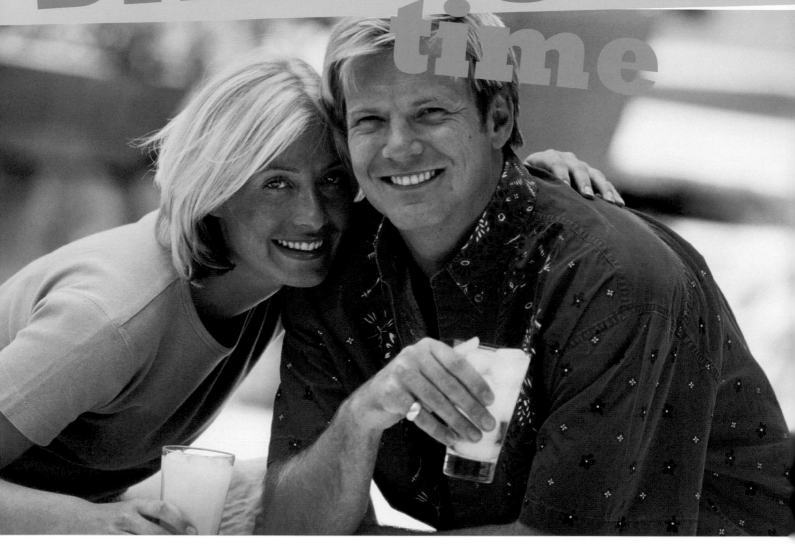

Are you someone who is used to having the odd drink each evening or who likes to go out with friends for a few? You may need to think about changing your lifestyle if you are planning to get pregnant. Our top tips will help you.

What's in a unit?

Even when you are not thinking about getting pregnant, it is an idea to keep an eye on how much you are drinking. Alcohol interferes with the way in which the body can take in vitamins and minerals. It also makes it harder for essential organs, such as the liver, to cope.

To help people know how much they can safely drink, advice is given in units per week. This does not mean that you can drink the whole amount for the week in one go! This type of 'binge' drinking is quite harmful because the body then has to work very hard to get rid of the poisons.

One unit of alcohol =

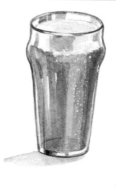
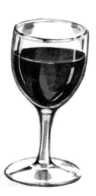

Begin by cutting down

You could start by cutting down the amount of alcohol you drink. Alcohol is measured in units. A small glass of wine is one unit so is half a pint of beer, lager or cider. These measures are the ones used in bars and pubs. Watch out at home though; most people pour a lot more than a standard measure!

Aim first of all to get down to seven units of alcohol spread across a week. This is the amount that women can safely have when they are not pregnant. Once you have cracked that as a target, try to cut down to two units a week. In the first twelve weeks try to avoid alcohol altogether if you can manage it.

1 Begin by proving to yourself that you don't need drink. See if you can spend a couple of days without drinking. This will give you a lot of confidence.

2 Encourage your partner to join in as cutting back makes a difference to men's fertility.

3 Try changing your routines. Some drinking can begin just as a habit. Go out to the cinema or have a pizza rather than go to places where it is hard to escape drinking.

4 Make sure that you have plenty of non-alcoholic drinks around at home. Look out for alcohol-free lager and wines, as well as some of the more interesting drinks such as ice cold teas, smoothies and sparkling water.

5 Choose long drinks and ask for plenty of the non-alcoholic ingredient mixer e.g. half a pint of shandy with a hint of lager or beer.

6 Avoid eating salty snack foods when you are out. These will make you more thirsty and more likely to want to drink more.

7 Offer to be the driver.

HONESTY
- a best policy?

Maybe you smoke, Maybe you drink. Maybe you do other stuff too. So what should you do when you see the doctor? We ask our health experts about just how honest you can be.

No one likes to admit that they are taking things that are bad for them or are downright illegal. After all, there are plenty of health messages around and most of us know what we should and shouldn't be doing. So, you may be tempted to keep quiet about needing a drink or having a little smoke to help you relax. While this may seem like the best option, you might be pleasantly surprised to find out that people working with pregnant women or those trying to get pregnant are on your side. 'Women sometimes think that they will be told off or given a hard time, but that's not what we are about,' says Penny, a midwife in Bristol 'At the end of the day, what we really want is for women to have healthy babies and to do that means working *with* women not against them.' This view is echoed over and over again by other health professionals who would far prefer women to be honest with them so that they can give the right kind of care, as Ian, a GP from Liverpool explains, 'Attitudes have changed a lot over the years. We now work with women and look at ways of helping them and their babies. To do this means that we need women to be ready to talk to us. Sadly, though that message still needs to be put across more.'

Don't be afraid – GPs, midwives and other health professionals are far more friendly and in touch than before. They are there to give you and your baby support.

See your doctor early on – The sooner that you get in contact, the more time there will be to plan your pregnancy.

Be honest – The more that your GP and midwife know, the easier it is for them to help you conceive or, if you are pregnant, to get the care of the baby right.

Attend your appointments – Once you get pregnant you will need to see your midwife or GP regularly. This way they can check on the progress of your baby and make sure that all is well. The aim of these visits is not to 'spy' on you, although they will obviously want to see that you are keeping well. Seeing the same GP or midwife will also help you feel more and more comfortable.

INFECTION ALERT

Germs in the form of viruses and bacteria are around us all the time. Some, which are harmless most of the time, can pose a threat to women who are pregnant or planning to conceive. Over the next few pages, we look at the infections you really need to know about.

CHILDHOOD INFECTIONS – NOT QUITE AS THEY SEEM

You may not have children or have regular contact with them, but childhood illnesses often do the rounds and so, even at a supermarket, you may be exposed to some common childhood illnesses.

Some common childhood infections are a bit like Jekyll and Hyde. On the surface they appear perfectly harmless, causing at the most some irritating symptoms, but catch them in pregnancy and the effects can be devastating. Knowing about the infections can help you to avoid them or take steps to prevent catching them.

Chicken Pox (varicella zoster)

Whoever would have thought that chicken pox would be a problem! Most people think of chicken pox as an unpleasant childhood illness which causes itchy spots that turn to scabs. Sadly though, chicken pox is far from harmless. While some children can get complications, pregnant women are very much at risk. If caught in the early weeks of pregnancy when the embryo is still forming the virus can cause a range of abnormalities. After the fourth month of pregnancy, the damage from the virus lessens, although if women catch it around the time that they give birth, complications can occur.

German measles (rubella)

German measles or rubella is quite a rare infection nowadays because most girls have already been vaccinated. Symptoms include a rash that starts on the face and spreads down to the chest, arms and legs. In itself, the infection is not serious, but if caught in early pregnancy the effects on the baby may be very serious and are known as the 'rubella syndrome'. The earlier on in pregnancy that the infection is contracted, the more severe the effects. These can include blindness and deafness in the baby, as well as possible miscarriage.

Slapped Cheek syndrome (erythrovirus type B19)

This is one that you may not have heard of, but is quite common in children. The infection gives children a red rash on their cheek – hence its name. It can sometimes be a problem in pregnancy, although fortunately it is quite rare. Its effects include miscarriage and stillbirth and some fetal deformities.

Essential steps

1. Find out whether or not you have already had chicken pox as a child. If so you should have some antibodies that will protect you. If you have not had chicken pox, your doctor may check your immunity and offer you a vaccination.
2. Avoid contact with children and adults who have either chicken pox or its cousin shingles. If you work with children, make sure that you tell your doctor before you become pregnant.
3. Once you are pregnant, if you have contact with someone who has the infection, make an appointment to see your doctor immediately.

Essential steps

1. Find out if you have been vaccinated against this disease. If you are not completely sure, it is essential to have your immunity checked by your doctor before you get pregnant. A simple blood test will confirm whether or not you are immune. A vaccination will then be offered.
2. If you are not rubella immune and are pregnant, contact your doctor if you think that you have come into contact with the disease. You may for example have been travelling abroad.

Essential steps

1. If possible, avoid being in contact with children with this infection.
2. If you know that you have been in contact with the disease, make an immediate appointment to see your family doctor.

Fact file ... Toxoplasmosis

Behind this big word is a tiny parasite that can do quite a bit of harm in pregnancy. We turn the spotlight on to understanding how this parasite goes about its business and how you can avoid catching it.

What is it?

Toxoplasmosis is a tiny parasite that is found in meat, cat's mess and also in soil where cats may have dirtied.

How can it be caught?

The parasite is usually taken in by swallowing something that has been infected with the parasite. It can be caught by humans as well as other animals and birds.

Why does it matter?

Most healthy people who get toxoplasmosis will probably never know it. The most usual symptom is a flu-like illness, although occasionally strong reactions can occur. Sadly in pregnancy, the effects of toxoplasmosis can be more severe and affect the unborn baby. In the first twelve weeks of pregnancy toxoplasmosis is at its most dangerous and can cause miscarriage or damage to the baby's brain and other organs. If caught later in pregnancy, it can still cause damage particularly to the baby's eyes.

IF YOU GET A FLU-LIKE ILLNESS IN PREGNANCY, CONTACT YOUR DOCTOR

Treatment for toxoplasmosis

Ideally, you should try to avoid contracting toxoplasmosis by following the steps in the chart below. If you feel that you are at risk or have flu-like symptoms, you should see a doctor immediately. A blood test will be carried out to assess whether or not you are already immune or have a current infection. Once the results of the test are back (which can take up to three weeks) your doctor will talk through what action if any needs taking. Happily, the effects of acute toxoplasmosis in pregnancy are quite rare as many women with an active infection do not pass it onto the unborn baby.

Practical steps to avoid toxoplasmosis

There are many practical ways in which you can avoid getting toxoplasmosis. Many of them will also prevent you from getting other diseases.

Fruit and vegetables

Wash your hands before preparing food.
Wash all fruit and vegetables thoroughly.
Wash chopping boards, knives and utensils after preparing the fruit and vegetables.

Outdoors

Wear gloves when gardening. Wash hands afterwards.
Cover children's sand boxes to prevent cats using them as litter trays.
Wash hands before eating even before having a picnic or eating an ice cream. Avoid contact with sheep and newborn lambs.

Meat

Wash hands before and after touching raw meat.
Wash chopping boards, knives and other utensils immediately after raw meat has touched them.
Eat only meat that has been thoroughly cooked through.
Avoid raw fish.
Avoid raw cured meats such as parma ham.

Cats and other animals

Wear gloves when changing litter trays or better still ask someone else to do it.
Wash hands after touching animals.
Check that your cat is in good health.
Avoid contact with sheep and new born lambs for example, don't visit a farm in spring time.

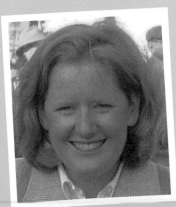

Most people have never heard of toxoplasmosis. Diana Brocklebank Scott was typical of many women. In February 2001 she was diagnosed as having acute toxoplasmosis and later lost her unborn baby.

'Before becoming pregnant, I had read a number of general leaflets about pre-pregnancy care but most focused on general diet. I had been given no advice about how to avoid getting toxoplasmosis. Soon after being diagnosed with it, I realised that information about the condition, and specifically awareness of its prevention, was lacking. 2001 was a difficult year for my husband, Anthony, and me; we lost our baby because of an infection that is preventable. Toxoplasmosis is detectable by a simple blood test, just like rubella. A healthy person who has had it carries the antibodies and is immune to further infection. Women who are immune protect their unborn children. However, women who are not immune can take simple precautions to avoid catching it.'

'We resolved to help Tommy's, the baby charity, to raise money to provide better information on toxoplasmosis. We wanted to target this information at those who are considering starting a family and to the wider public. Anthony and four of our friends, Alan Kasket, Stuart Grant, Ivo Clifton and Jenny Robins, formed 'Team Toxo' and ran the gruelling 26.2 miles of the 2002 London Marathon, raising £63,836 for Tommy's.'

SEXUALLY TRANSMITTED INFECTIONS –
could it be you?

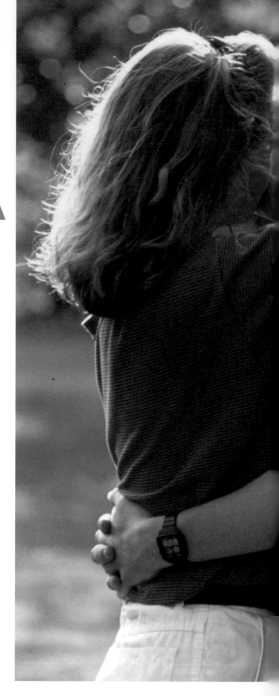

Sexually transmitted infections are back and very much on the increase. They are can be the reason behind infertility and miscarriage, although many have few if any symptoms. Our special report looks at what is out there and whether you could be at risk.

In the UK the days when men and women were virgins on their wedding night are long gone. These days most women and men spend some time enjoying sexual freedom before settling down. While few people want to go back to the chaste old days, it is a fact of life that sexually transmitted infections (STIs) are on the increase, as Maria Simpson explains. 'While most people are aware of the HIV/AIDS message, we have seen a huge increase in other STIs over the past few years. Most worrying is perhaps chlamydia which is now the commonest bacterial infection.'

'Chlamydia is easily treatable if caught early on'

Health professionals say chlamydia is a huge concern because of its ability to leave women infertile without them necessarily having any symptoms. Maria explains, 'Chlamydia has been on the increase and although some women may get some vaginal discharge, many others will not.

It is a progressive disease and if it reaches the fallopian tubes can cause scarring and infertility. The good news, however, is that it is easily treatable with antibiotics if caught early on. Our advice to women is always to come in regularly and get screened particularly if they have had a recent change of partner or know that at one time in their lives they may have been at risk.'

'They may have moved on emotionally, but the STI stays around'

When it comes to who may be at risk, it can be anyone who has had several sexual relationships and not always used condoms.' STIs are a fact of life rather than a stigma. We see men and women from every walk of life. Sometimes they realise that they have picked up an infection from a previous partner's partner. The message to couples is to use condoms until they are completely sure that neither they nor their partner has been at risk in the past. It's easy for couples to forget past behaviour and relationships once they are committed to a relationship. Sadly, while they may have moved on emotionally, the STI stays around.' Maria reminds couples that if their relationship is stable and they are thinking of starting a family, it might be a good time to talk honestly about their previous histories. 'We have had women whose partners have had one night stands in the past and the first time that they find out there is any problem is when they can't conceive.'

'Being screened for infection can be a good idea'

So when and where should you go for help? Maria suggests it can be a good idea to have a health check up before trying for a baby, if women know that they or their partner may at some time have been at risk. She explains that the best place to go is the health centre or professional clinic where you feel comfortable. She also emphasises that all information is confidential and screening for specific infections only takes place with consent.

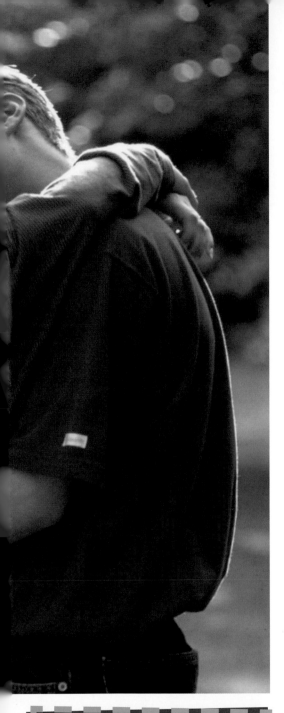

What's out there?

This table shows

Name	Female symptoms	Male symptoms	Treatment
Chlamydia	Vaginal discharge. Pain or burning sensation when passing urine. Not all women have symptoms.	Unusual discharge, soreness or other symptoms. Can lead to lower sperm count, lower sperm motility and more abnormal sperm.	Early treatment with antibiotics.
Gonorrhoea	Vaginal discharge. Pain or burning sensation when passing urine. Painful abdomen.	Unusual discharge. Pain or burning sensation when passing urine. Irritation of the penis. Redness at the opening of the urethra at the end of the penis.	Early treatment with antibiotics.
Herpes	Painful blisters on genitals. Pain when urinating.	Painful blisters on genitals.	Ointment. Do not have oral sex with anyone who has cold sores.
Hepatitis B	Some or all of the following: flu-like symptoms (cough, sore throat), tiredness, mild fever, muscle and joint aches, loss of appetite, nausea, vomiting.	Some or all of the following: flu-like symptoms (cough, sore throat), tiredness, mild fever, muscle and joint aches, loss of appetite, nausea, vomiting.	No treatment, but rest and good food can aid recovery after a few months. Vaccine available for people who are at risk of catching it e.g. travellers, health workers.
HIV	No symptoms for many years but can develop into AIDS which is life-threatening.	No symptoms for many years but can develop into AIDS which is life-threatening. A new technique, where semen is 'washed', can allow HIV-positive men to father healthy children without increasing the risk of infecting an HIV-negative partner.	No cure, but treatments available. Health workers and people who travel in some other countries should take preventative measures. Women with known infection can be helped to have a safe pregnancy and birth.

SEEK HELP IF YOU:
Have pain during or after sex
Notice a change in
vaginal discharge
Have pain or feel stinging
when urinating
Spot blood in between
your periods
Have any blisters on genitals
Begin to have heavy periods

Could you be at risk?

It is easy to want to forget past behaviour that may have been risky, but look at these questions with your partner to assess whether either of you might be at risk.

1 Were you sexually active or did you have several partners between the ages of 16-24?

2 Have you or your partner had unprotected sex on a one-night stand or on a holiday?

3 Have you had a recent change of partner?

4 Have you or your partner had anal sex without a condom?

5 Have you or your partner ever had a sexually transmitted infection?

6 Have you or your partner ever used needles to take drugs?

7 Have you been in a relationship with a partner who has travelled abroad?

8 Do you have any concerns that your partner has been unfaithful at any time in your relationship?

9 Have either of you had more than four sexual partners in your lives?

10 Have you ever had bleeding between periods?

11 Have you have pain or a burning sensation in passing urine?

12 Have you ever had painful sexual intercourse?

13 Do you have very heavy periods?

14 Have you ever had oral sex while you or your partner has had a cold sore on the mouth?

15 Do you use sex toys anally and vaginally?

If you can answer yes to one or more of these questions, it might be worth getting yourself checked out as a precautionary measure. Make an appointment either with your practice nurse, GP, family planning or genital urinary clinic. Go where you feel most comfortable.

Are there aspects of your lifestyle that could be important to think about when trying for a baby?

We've got all the information for you here!

Many infections do not have the same effects throughout life as they do if caught during pregnancy. To find out how to protect yourself check out these pages.

INFECTION **ALERT**

pages 52/53

Could you be at risk from a sexually transmitted infection? Many people in the UK are and may not even realise it. Try our quiz and find out more.

Could you be at risk?

page 56

Stopping smoking has an enormous impact on the potential health of a growing baby – if you'd like to know more about how to give up take a look at our tips and the different support that is available for you.

Saying farewell to smoking

pages 63–65

LOOK GOOD, FEEL GOOD!

Everyone knows that a little bit of exercise is good for us. But how should you go about it, if you have always been a couch potato? We ask our exercise and fitness expert Judy Di Fiore to give us a few tips.

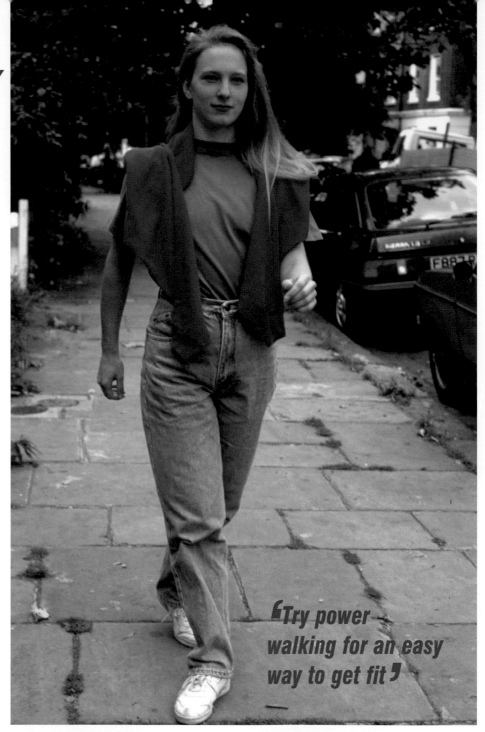

'Try power walking for an easy way to get fit'

Being reasonably fit is not a bad thing if you are thinking about starting a family or launching into another pregnancy as Judy explains, 'Pregnancy can put a lot of strain on the body and can be tiring. If you have the correct balance of muscular strength and flexibility, you can cope more easily with the demands of pregnancy.' Judy also explains that being in good shape can also help you conceive in the first place. 'The body works more efficiently when you're fit and being toned up usually makes you feel more confident about yourself.'

In addition to helping you to conceive and cope with the pregnancy, Judy is keen to point out other spin offs. 'Some very simple exercises will help you to tone up, lose weight and make you look great.'

START WITH POSTURE

Judy suggests that a good start is the change of weight/balance and think about your posture. 'This is one of the most important aspects of pregnancy as changing posture can put a lot of pressure on the back and many women get backache. Correct body alignment will strengthen essential postural muscles.' To start with Judy has some very simple suggestions. 'Begin by being aware of the way in which you sit and stand. Aim not to crumple into a sofa, but to sit with a cushion behind so you can be more upright.' Judy also suggests that by having good posture when you walk, you can also look slimmer. 'Women should try and walk tall, without tucking their bottoms in'. For those of us who try and breathe in to hold our stomachs in and push our bottoms in, Judy has a word of caution. 'Holding your breath or squeezing your bottom in actually takes the spine out of its correct alignment and this can create postural problems.'

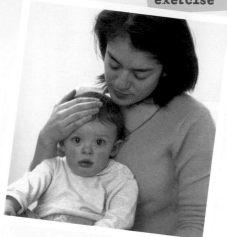

TUMMY IN

Looking slimmer doesn't mean doing hundreds of sit ups as these will not flatten your tummy. Judy recommends a simple exercise which will flatten your tummy and help to support the all-important lower back. This exercise involves drawing your tummy button in towards your spine. 'The trick is to pull your tummy in without holding your breath or raising your shoulders' explains Judy 'it's a good idea to try it whilst talking so that you cannot hold your breath. If women aim to do it five times a day, they will quickly build muscles and find that their posture, and lower back discomfort improves.'

STEPPING OUT

As well as looking at posture, Judy also recommends building up cardiovascular fitness. 'Ideally women need to be in good shape before they get pregnant. This will help them to cope with the heavy demands of pregnancy and help them to get back into shape afterwards. She suggests that you can begin by walking up and down the stairs instead of taking the lift or escalator. This is apparently brilliant to shape up bottoms and to tone the legs. 'Women can start by walking up and down stairs three times a week and then increase the amount they are doing. Most women are surprised how easy this then becomes.' Judy has some interesting tips as to how to start off. 'You can build up your walking stamina by getting off a bus one stop early or parking the car a little further away so as to walk further. Once people

begin to walk, they soon find it becomes easier and easier.' The next step can be to graduate into a slightly more strenuous walk known as power walking. 'Power walking is an excellent type of cardiovascular exercise. Take long strides, driving your heels into the floor and pushing off with the ball of the foot. Swing your arms by your sides and walk at a brisk pace.'

OUT AND ABOUT

For those of you who are inspired to go one step further and get really fit, but who do not want to go to the gym, Judy offers some alternatives. 'Getting fit does not have to mean going to a smart club and working out. Belly dancing, salsa classes and line dancing are all ways in which activity levels can be raised.' Judy is keen to reassure those of us who feel a bit self conscious too. 'Leisure centres tend to have mixed ability classes so that you can start off as a beginner and wear comfortable, baggy clothing. Judy is also keen to emphasise that enjoyment is important. 'It's always better to do something that you enjoy because that way you are likely to keep it up. Going out to a class with a few friends and having a laugh is a great way of getting your body back into shape.' Judy also has some thoughts if you are overweight. 'Increasing activity is a fantastic way of losing weight, but people who are very overweight may need to begin by walking rather than jogging or running. Gentle exercise such as walking, swimming and aqua aerobics are great because they do not put pressure on the joints.'

Experts tell us that exercise can make a real difference not only during pregnancy but also before and after. Ramoni, with Marco 4 years and now Arianna 6 months knows from her personal experience what a difference some simple exercises made.

'The first time round with Marco, I didn't do any exercise at all. Not before, during or even after the pregnancy. I just thought that once you had a baby, your body goes back to normal. It was a real shock when it didn't work that way. I felt like a balloon and my tummy was all floppy. After a few months, I also put on weight. I was so unhappy at the way I looked; I ended up eating more to make me feel better. Marco wasn't an easy baby and as well as feeling miserable about the way I looked, I also was tired. To cap it all, I also had times when I was incontinent.

With Arianne, it was completely different. I had already started some exercise classes and was beginning to feel that I had my body back under my control. I had also met some other friends and so when I found out I was pregnant, I was determined to make sure that I stayed in shape. I didn't do anything that was energetic, but just made sure that I worked on my posture and exercised gently. With some of the exercises, such as pulling in your tummy, I could also do them at home. I remember sweeping the floor and reminding myself to pull in! The difference it made was incredible. The pregnancy went more smoothly and I had more energy and strength. With Marco, I had back pains and sciatica and felt quite heavy. The best bit was seeing how quickly I got my shape back after the birth. Instead of feeling like a balloon, I felt happy because I not only had a lovely baby but I also had my body back.'

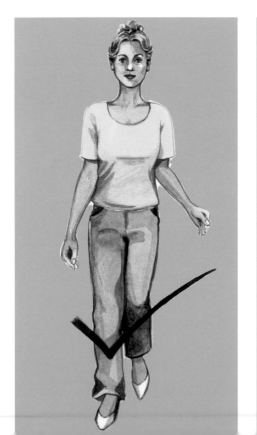

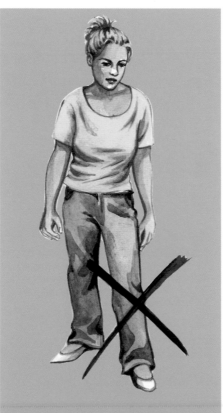

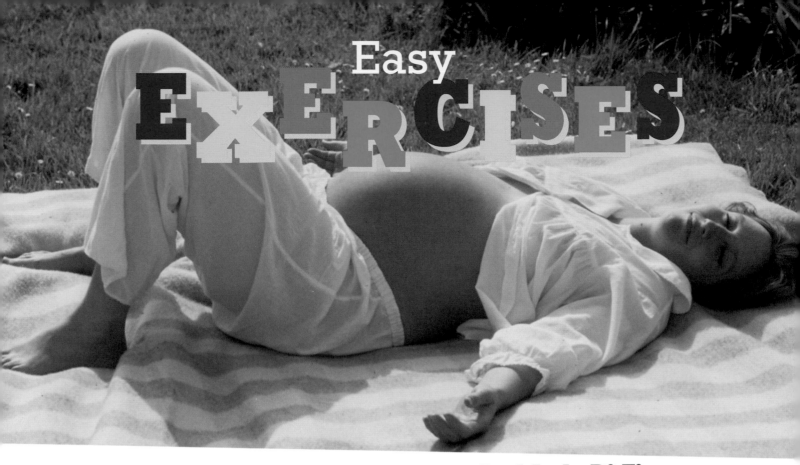

Easy EXERCISES

To help you on your way, we have asked Judy Di Fiore a specialist consultant in Ante/Postnatal Fitness to give us two exercises that will tone and trim.

Bridge

This exercise is great for loosening stiff backs and also strengthens the abdominal muscles.

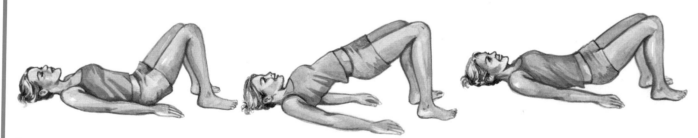

1 Lie on your back with knees bent up and feet flat on the floor, arms relaxed by your sides

2 Draw your tummy in and roll your pelvis so the pubic bone lifts and the lower back presses into the floor. Continue the movement upwards by lifting the bottom and rolling the spine slowly off the floor, one vertebra at a time until the tips of the shoulder blades are lifted off the floor. Pause for a few seconds trying not to grip too tightly with the buttocks

3 Keeping the buttocks lifted until the last moment, lower the back slowly down to the floor, one vertebra at a time. Use your abdominal muscles to control the movement.

Pelvic floor

**A must for everyone – these muscles support your internal organs which get stretched during pregnancy.
By keeping them strong, you will stop yourself from wetting yourself when you cough, sneeze or laugh.
You need to practise both the slow and the fast exercises as often as possible.**

1 Slow exercise

Slowly tighten the muscles around your back and front passages, as if to stop yourself going to the loo, and feel them lift them up inside you. Hold for a few seconds continuing to breathe then release with control.

2 Fast exercise

As number 1 with one quick tightening action and release immediately, with control.

Judy has written two books:
The Pregnancy Exercise Book
Judy DiFiore (Newleaf 2000) £9.99 + p&p

The Complete Guide to Postnatal Fitness
Judy DiFiore (A & C Black 1998) £13.99 + p&p

Hints to healthy exercising

Begin by increasing your activity level gradually

Start off by walking more or joining some kind of a beginner's exercise class. Remember that any extra increase in activity can only do some good.

Set yourself small but achievable targets

Many people make the mistake of trying to do more than they can really manage. This means that they quickly lose heart and give up. Try to give yourself easy targets and then keep building them up. Remember that small and regular bouts of exercise are better than the odd hour once a month.

Look for activities that you find enjoyable

Getting fit should not make you feel miserable. Activities such as badminton, swimming as well as yoga, pilates, belly dancing or even line dancing will all increase your overall activity level. You are far more likely to keep fit if you enjoy what you are doing.

Enlist the help of a work colleague, friend or partner

Some people feel that they don't have the time to get fit. Try seeing if you can do something at lunch time or encourage your partner to go for a walk or join a class with you.

Don't worry about the way you look

You do not need sportswear to do most types of exercise. Look out for comfortable baggy clothes rather than squeezing into lycra!

Avoid over-straining muscles

Many people think that they should feel pain as they exercise. This is not true. You should feel that you have exercised, but not be stiff or uncomfortable. Over-straining muscles can lead to injuries.

Don't have a large meal before exercising

It's much harder to get your body going if you have eaten a lot before doing any kind of exercise. Have a light, healthy snack if you are desperate for something to eat beforehand.

Make sure that you are wearing suitable shoes

It is a good idea to wear flat comfortable shoes for walking, while you will need a proper pair of trainers for other types of exercise such as jogging or aerobic classes. Choose trainers that have cushioned soles rather than ones that are made for casual wear. Ask your sports shop or an instructor at a leisure centre for some advice if you are not sure.

Take some water with you

Ideally, your exercise should make you just slightly breathless. This means that your heart and lungs are working a little harder than usual. You may find that you feel thirsty afterwards and so take some water with you. Avoid alcohol at all costs. Not only will it pile on the weight, it will also dehydrate you.

Take some healthy snacks for afterwards

Many people feel hungry after they have exercised. Avoid high energy drinks and snacks if you are also trying to lose a little weight. Carry with you some healthy snacks such as a banana, apple, cereal bar etc.

To SMOKE or not to SMOKE

You may have tried to stop smoking or you may just be thinking about it. We look at the facts behind smoking and some of the ways and aids to stop smoking.

Smoking: Your life – Your choice

If you are a smoker, you may feel under attack from adverts, family and even your doctor. So what's the big deal? At the end of the day, you can only give up smoking if you want to. This means making a choice. But you can only make this choice if you have the information. We provide you with the information that you need.

Fact 1

It may seem incredible, but smoke contains over 4000 different chemicals. These add up to a poisonous cocktail.

Fact 2

Cigarettes contain nicotine. Nicotine makes your heart beat faster and gives an instant 'lift'. This is why you may enjoy smoking. Unfortunately you can get addicted to nicotine, which is why smoking is so difficult to give up.

Fact 3

Cigarette smoke contains carbon monoxide. After a while, it starves your body of oxygen and damages your lungs and blood vessels.

Fact 4

Because smoking affects the amount of blood and oxygen that can get through to the unborn baby, many babies whose mother's smoke are born underweight and early. In some cases, smoking is a factor in stillbirth. Babies who are premature or underweight cannot always go home with their mothers after the birth because they need extra medical attention.

Fact 5

It's not just women who are affected by smoking. Smoking can actually damage men's sperm lowering their sperm count.

Fact 6

Because smoking affects the amount of oxygen available in our bodies, it is harder for cells to be repaired and maintained. This is why skin ages more in smokers and why they are more prone to infections.

Fact 7

Babies whose parents smoke are at a higher risk of cot death. There are a number of reasons for this, but they all link back to reduced oxygen levels. Even holding a baby after you have smoked can reduce their oxygen levels.

Fact 8

Children who see their parents smoke are more likely to become smokers themselves. The old expression 'do as I say, not as I do' comes to mind here! Giving up before your child is born means that you will be giving them a good chance of being free of the weed.

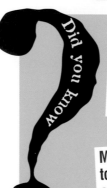
Did you know

Stopping smoking when you are pregnant makes an almost immediate difference to your baby. One study showed that after just 48 hours, unborn babies were getting up to 8% more oxygen.

More people die through smoking tobacco than through taking any other legal or illegal drug.

Saying farewell to smoking

– SOME PRACTICAL TIPS

1 PLAN AHEAD

Research shows that people who plan ahead are more likely to succeed in giving up cigarettes. Choose a time when you aren't under stress and give yourself a start date. If you have already tried and failed in the past to give up, think about what made you go back to smoking. Aim to stop this from happening again.

2 LEARN ABOUT YOUR SMOKING HABIT

Think about the situations in which you smoke. Keep a smoking diary so that you can see when you are in the habit of smoking. Go on to the www.givingupsmoking.co.uk website to see how addicted you are to nicotine. As a broad rule of thumb, if you smoke more than 10 cigarettes a day and desperately need a cigarette first thing in the morning you will find it hard to give up without some sort of support such as nicotine replacement patches.

3 GET ALL THE HELP YOU CAN

See your doctor about nicotine replacement therapy (NRT) patches or gum. These are now available on prescription. Find out about smoking cessation clinics and also other sources of support such as www.givingupsmoking.co.uk. Write the number of the NHS smoking helpline on all telephones (0800 169 0 169). Tell friends and family that you are giving up get them to help and support you.

4 REMOVE POSSIBLE REMINDERS IN YOUR HOME

It is much harder to give up if you can see and smell things that remind you of smoking. Take away ashtrays, clean rooms thoroughly to remove smoke smells.

5 KEEP REMINDING YOURSELF WHY YOU ARE TRYING TO GIVE UP

Write down all the good reasons for giving up – looking better, more money, no more cravings.

6 AVOID SITUATIONS WHICH MAY BE DIFFICULT

Work out where you are most likely to fall back into smoking. This may be with certain friends or when you are bored. Think about what you could do to change the situation. If you are not sure about when you smoke, try keeping a smoking diary before you give up. This will help you to identify times when you smoke.

7 WHEN YOU GET THE URGE TO SMOKE, FIND SOMETHING ELSE TO DO INSTEAD

Phone a friend, the NHS helpline and try to do something else with your hands and mouth. Some ex-smokers use chewing gum, suck lollipops or occupy their hands with worry beads. It has even been known for people to take up knitting.

8 SET TARGETS AND REWARD YOURSELF IF YOU REACH THEM.

If you haven't smoked for a week you could use the money you have saved to buy something really nice for yourself.

9 DON'T GIVE UP EVEN IF YOU HAVE A LAPSE

If you have a cigarette, don't feel that all is lost and there's no point in going on. Every time that you can manage without smoking is a victory in itself. Try to work out what caused you to slip-up and think of strategies to cope with this when it happens in the future.

10 IF YOU CAN'T GIVE UP, TRY CUTTING DOWN

For some people stopping smoking completely does not work. Try cutting down on the number of cigarettes you smoke instead and build up the number of hours that you can manage without a cigarette especially first thing in the morning. Switch to the lowest brand possible that you can. Consider having some rooms that are smoke free.

SMOKING

Once you have decided to give up smoking, it is a good idea to be aware of the support available and ways of going about giving up. We look at the variety of methods that may help you to quit.

Nicotine Replacement Therapy (NRT)

What is it?
Nicotine replacement therapy comes in different forms. You can get gum, patches, nasal sprays and microtabs.

How does it work?
Nicotine replacement therapy contains small amounts of nicotine. It works by reducing the withdrawal symptoms and can prevent you from having strong cravings.

Which NRT product should I use?
Different products work in slightly different ways and so it is a good idea to get some advice as to which will work best for you. If you are pregnant or have a medical condition, talk to your doctor and check that you can use these products.

- **Patches** worn on the arm release steady doses throughout the day and night.
- **Nasal sprays** give a strong instant dose of nicotine and are usually used by very heavy smokers.
- **Gum** is chewed and then put onto the cheek of the mouth so that the nicotine is absorbed through the gum. Gum allows you to control your nicotine dose.
- **Microtabs** are popped under the tongue when you have a craving and gradually dissolve.

Does it work?
It is very popular and has been shown to help people who really want to give up. Some research shows that people who use NRT to help them give up smoking are twice as likely to succeed as those who don't.

Where can I get it from?
You can buy NRT products in chemists, but your doctor can also give it to you on prescription.

Cold turkey

What is it?
Going cold turkey means stopping smoking completely and not replacing the nicotine. Cigarettes contain nicotine which is an extremely addictive substance. When your body craves a cigarette, it is actually looking to get nicotine.

How does it work?
Cold turkey literally means stopping smoking altogether. This means that the body has to cope without any nicotine.

Does it work?
Success can be very variable. Many people do give up this way, but success depends very much on willpower and also the strength of your addiction. The physical cravings for nicotine can carry on for 2-3 weeks and so 'cold turkey' without any other form of support can be very hard going.

Smoking cessation clinics

What are they?
Smoking cessation clinics are also called 'Stop smoking' clinics. They are often held in GPs surgeries or health clinics but are also in some hospitals.

How does it work?
Smoking cessation clinics work by giving practical advice and support to smokers. The idea is to help smokers find ways to stop smoking and to provide information that will help. Patients are usually encouraged to attend weekly and may as part of their visit discuss any difficulties they are having including the odd lapse. The nurses or health professionals running the clinics are very sympathetic and look at ways to help smokers to manage their addiction.

Does it work?
Many smokers find the weekly visit very useful as part of an overall plan to give up smoking. Success at the end of the day is not guaranteed, but research shows that where smokers are being supported, they are more likely to succeed.

Where can I get it from?
Either contact your doctor's surgery or phone the NHS smoking helpline on 0800 169 0169. Sessions are free.

Acupuncture

What is it?
Acupuncture is a Chinese method of healing which has been used for many centuries.

How does it work?
Needles are inserted at particular points in the body to cause patients to relax. Surprisingly, people who try this method do not find it painful. The needles are then removed, but two or three are sometimes left in the ear lobe. Patients are then encouraged to touch these when a craving comes on.

Does it work?
Some people find this method very effective, although it is not clinically proven.

Where can I get it from?
You are likely to have to pay for acupuncture sessions. The cost of each session can vary according to each practitioner. Find an acupuncturist through a recommendation if possible. Make sure that the acupuncturist is a member of either the British Medical Acupuncture Society (tel 01925 730727, website www.medical-acupuncture.co.uk) or the British Acupuncture Council (tel 020 8735 0400, website www.acupuncture.org.uk).

Hypnotherapy

What is it?
Hypnotherapy is a treatment that works on the subconscious mind. No drugs are taken.

How does it work?
Many people have not only a physical addiction to smoking but also a psychological one. Smoking cigarettes can be a way of coping with stressful situations or provide you with pleasant memories. Hypnotherapy works by giving your subconscious new messages about smoking.

Does it work?
Hypnotherapy is gaining in popularity. Some ex-smokers, swear by it, although there is no guarantee that it will work for you.

Where can I get it from?
The chances are that you will need to see a hynotherapist privately and pay for your consultation. Prices range from area to area. To choose a hypnotherapist, look for recommendations from friends or people that you know who have found it helpful. Hynotherapists advertise their services in a range of places such as Yellow Pages, health food shops or local papers. Check that your hypnotherapist is qualified and a member of a professional organisation such as the British Society of Clinical Hypnosis (tel 01262 403103, website fmp.bsch.org.uk) or registered with the British Hypnotherapy Association (tel 020 7723 4443).

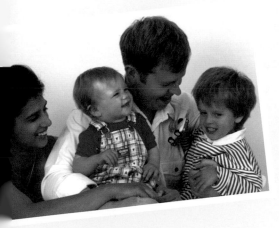

Third time lucky!!

Linda 30 and her partner Barry have two children, Niamh aged 2 years and Ben 15 months.

Linda and Barry gave up smoking before she became pregnant with Niamh. She had two failed attempts at stopping smoking before she finally cracked it.

'When I talked about having children with Barry, he was clear that he didn't want us to start a family until I had stopped smoking. His sister's baby had died of cot death and he had read that it was more likely to happen where the parents had smoked.

My first attempt only lasted three days. Looking back, I can see why it didn't work. Smoking was part of my life since I was eighteen years old and when I met Barry and tried giving up, I was probably smoking around thirty cigarettes a day. He didn't know how many I was smoking because if he asked, I would always knock off a few because I knew that he didn't like me smoking. When I first stopped smoking, Barry was so pleased for me. He bought me a little present each day to help me. I thought that I could do it, but the cravings were awful. In the end, one morning when Barry had left for work, I went round to a neighbour who I hardly knew and asked for a cigarette. That really was the end of that attempt, because once I had started to smoke, I couldn't face going without again. I told myself that a few wouldn't really matter and that after all it was my life and my health. It was awful telling Barry because he so wanted me to stop and he so wanted to help me. The second time I gave up, I lasted longer and after the first attempt I was smoking a bit less anyway. I had found out about the Nicotine gum and was a little more prepared. I did quite well and got to nearly a month without anything. It was something

stupid that got me going again and afterwards I was really cross with myself. I had a bad day at work and went out for a drink with a friend. I then got a call to say that my gran wasn't well. I was upset and stressed and suddenly I felt that I couldn't cope unless I had a cigarette. It was like a part of me was looking for an excuse to start again and here it was. The worst bit was telling Barry because he was so sure that I had got over it. The good thing about the second attempt was that I had seen that I could manage to get over the first weeks and so if I had done it once, I could do it again. The second attempt also made me more determined to crack it. Quite quickly, I had noticed that food tasted really good and I just generally felt more alive.

A few weeks later, I gave up again. I was more ready than ever before. I visited my doctor who gave me Nicotine patches and I also went every week to the stop smoking clinic at the surgery. They were brilliant and really helped me to keep going. Barry helped me by making sure that the house was clear of ashtrays and together we tried to do new things together so that my routine was different. I put the money I was saving into a bank account and mentally thought of it as my baby fund! After six months, I knew that I had cracked it and soon after I fell pregnant with Niamh. I don't regret giving up. It wasn't easy, but I would do anything for my kids and knowing that this gave them a better start in life makes me feel quite proud of myself.'

Q. Help! I'm already pregnant and I still smoke. Am I harming my baby?

A. The sooner you can give up or cut right down the better. While not wanting to scare you, it is only fair that you understand that smoking does put babies at risk.

Ask your doctor for advice; you may be able to go on a short course of NRT or start visiting your local stop smoking clinic. If you continue to smoke during the pregnancy, look at ways of reducing the risk.
(see box below)

Q. I've tried giving up smoking before, but it has never worked. What should I do?

A. Don't beat yourself around the head with guilt. Guilt can actually make you smoke more! Many people need more than one attempt before they finally break the habit. The key to finally giving up is to plan your attempt and in the meantime to cut back. There is now plenty of support and advice around to help would-be quitters. Think about visiting your GP or phoning the NHS Smoking helpline on 0800 169 0 169 for advice .

Q. I want to give up smoking, but don't want to put on weight

A. Smoking affects people's taste buds and so food doesn't have the same taste. It also means that instead of nibbling when you are bored, you have something else in your mouth. Many people think that they will automatically put on weight when they stop smoking, but this does not have to be the case. Buy in lots of fresh fruit and dried raisins, prunes and even carrot sticks. You will find that these suddenly taste better because your taste buds can now pick up the flavours. If you need something to put in your mouth because you are missing cigarettes, try chewing sugar-free gum.

Q. I have heard that Zyban is worth trying. Where can I get hold of it?

A. Zyban also known as buproprion is a new drug and is only available on prescription. It is thought to be an effective treatment especially if it is taken alongside a smoking plan. It does have some side effects and so is not prescribed for everyone. It is not suitable for women who are pregnant or people with epilepsy. This may mean that if you are trying for a baby, your doctor will not prescribe it for you.

Last word if you have to smoke...

Smoking is definitely not safe. If you decide that you do not want to give up, there are a few things that you can do to make smoking a little safer. While this advice cannot guarantee that you will have a healthy pregnancy, it is worth following as even cutting down the amount you smoke will make a difference to a developing baby.

- Switch to low tar cigarettes.
- Do not smoke down to the filter. Try and leave the longest stub you can as this will reduce the amount of chemicals you are taking in.
- Cut down to five cigarettes a day.
- Try not to smoke one cigarette straight after another, otherwise you will always be looking for the next one.
- Avoid getting into the habit of smoking and drinking at the same time. It makes giving one or the other up, or cutting back, much harder.
- Stick to tobacco. Avoid other drugs such as cocaine or cannabis.
- Do not smoke around babies and make their bedrooms smoke-free zones.

Sadly, many things to do with pregnancy can go wrong, and many couples experiences difficulties before or during a pregnancy. If this is you, then you are not alone. Read on to find out more …

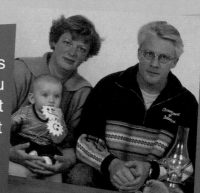

If you have experienced a pregnancy loss or miscarriage as so many couples do, then you may like to read other couples' stories about overcoming these complications and anxieties, or what you can do too reduce the risks of it happening again.

69–71
pages

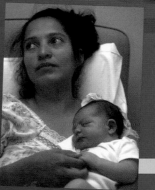

Perhaps genetics has always been an area you don't feel you understand, now's an opportunity for you to find out more through our "It's all in the genes" section.

76
page

Or if you have a history of illness or disease and wonder whether genetic counselling might be the answer, why not take a look at our feature.

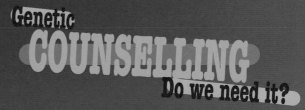
Genetic
COUNSELLING
Do we need it?

77
page

Infertility can be an area of great concern for many men and women, if you want to know more about what can be wrong and what can be done, this item might have the answer.

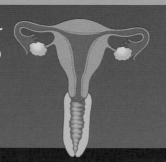

72/73
pages

Looking for a happy ending
THE STORY BEHIND MISCARRIAGES

IT IS A SAD FACT OF LIFE THAT NOT ALL PREGNANCIES GO SMOOTHLY. MISCARRIAGES AND STILLBIRTHS REMIND US THAT WE CAN'T COMPLETELY CONTROL MOTHER NATURE. OVER THE NEXT FEW PAGES, WE EXPLORE THE CAUSES OF MISCARRIAGE AND SOME OF THE WAYS IN WHICH WOMEN CAN SOMETIMES REDUCE THE ODDS OF HAVING ONE.

Talk to most couples who have children and you will probably find that either they or friends that they know have had a miscarriage. Miscarriages are quite common. It is thought that as many as one in five pregnancies will come to an early end. This may seem an alarming statistic, but it is not so bleak as at first sight. Firstly, many miscarriages occur even before a woman realises that she is pregnant and usually in the very first few days and weeks following conception. Stillbirth, the loss of an unborn baby after six months, is mercifully rare. Secondly, while of no immediate comfort at the time of a miscarriage or stillbirth, most women do go onto have a successful pregnancy next time.

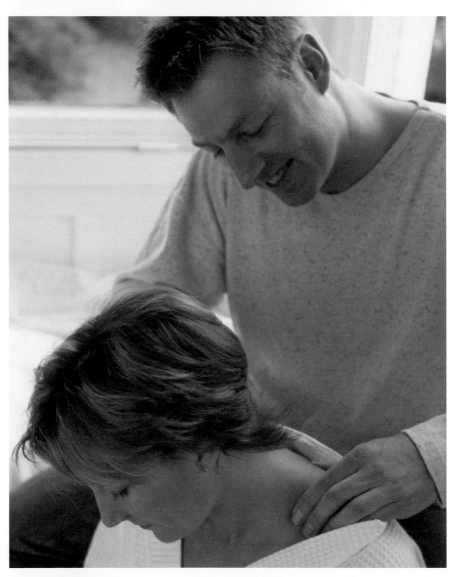

ALWAYS SEEK MEDICAL ADVICE IMMEDIATELY IF YOU HAVE ANY OF THE FOLLOWING SYMPTOMS:

Light bleeding or spotting

Strong abdominal pains

High fever

Heavy bleeding

MISSING INFORMATION – A COMMON CAUSE

'Why' is the biggest question that most couples want answering when a miscarriage happens. Sadly, many will never know as unless the woman suffers repeated miscarriage investigations are not often carried out. This is because miscarriages and stillbirths are often out of our immediate control. By far the commonest reason for miscarriage has to do with the genetic make up of the fertilised egg or the failure of the fertilised egg to implant itself correctly in the uterus.

It is thought that around half of all miscarriages are caused because at the moment of conception vital genetic information was either damaged or not present. The missing or damaged information means that the fetus can no longer carry on developing and naturally the pregnancy comes to an end.

THE WRONG PLACE

For a pregnancy to succeed, in the days after conception, the fertilised egg needs to implant itself properly into the lining of the uterus. Sometimes all does not go to plan. In some cases, the uterus is not correctly shaped or ready to receive the fertilised egg while in others the fertilised egg does not position itself correctly. Occasionally a fertilised egg will attach itself into a fallopian tube rather than go down into the uterus. This is called an ectopic pregnancy and is often characterised by intense abdominal pain which may result in an operation to remove part of the fallopian tube.

KNOWING THAT A MISCARRIAGE HAS TAKEN PLACE

Many women who have a very early miscarriage will never know for sure, as the only sign will be a slightly later period than expected and some heavier bleeding. For women who have a miscarriage later the early signs can vary. Some women report that they stop feeling pregnant, while for others the sign is the bleeding that begins to take place. It is important here to realise that not all pregnancies where bleeding takes place will automatically end in a miscarriage. Surprisingly, many women have spotting and bleeding in the early weeks of pregnancy particularly around the time of missed periods at 8 and 12 weeks. As it can be hard to know what is happening, seeking medical advice is always a good idea.

Once bleeding begins to take place, it can vary. Some women bleed continually and heavily for several days passing blood clots, others may bleed on and off. If doctors are concerned that any material from the pregnancy is left inside, women are offered a minor operation to clear the womb and to prevent a later infection.

TREATMENT FOLLOWING MISCARRIAGE

Most women are disappointed to find that investigation or treatment is not offered to them if it is their first or even second miscarriage. This is because most miscarriages are random and only in a few cases will women find that miscarriages keep occurring. Once a third miscarriage has taken place, however, women are usually referred for investigations to take place.

STARTING AGAIN

Couples vary in the time they wish to start trying for another pregnancy. Some couples want to try at once while others feel the need to grieve the loss. In pure physical terms, it is thought best if women wait for their next period before trying to conceive. This can take up to six weeks and gives the body time to recover physically.

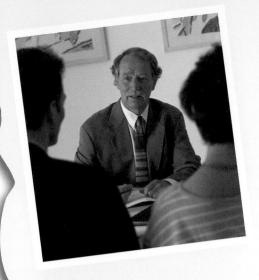

Hazel and Steve now have two children. Hazel's first pregnancy ended at 11 weeks.

'I remember walking through a park about a week before and realising that I didn't feel pregnant any more. It was my first pregnancy and to be honest, I didn't know what to expect. A week later I felt some dull cramps. It felt like period pains. Again, I wasn't really worried but did phone a midwife who told me to lie down. So I went off to bed, but later in the night I started to bleed. It was light at first, but I woke Steve and got him to phone the doctor. We were told to go the hospital. They were kind enough at the hospital, but I remember thinking that they were not in a hurry. I thought that they should be trying to stop the bleeding. Of course, I now know that they couldn't do anything, but I didn't know that then. After a while, I had a scan. It showed that the sac was empty and it confirmed that I was having a miscarriage. I was bleeding quite heavily. They kept me in overnight and I had a D and C. The next day, a really nice doctor told us that miscarriages were quite common and not to blame ourselves. He actually made me smile through my tears by saying that humans were not the best species when it came to reproduction and that luck had quite a lot to do with it. This made us both feel better and it did stop me from feeling guilty. I had wondered whether I had done something to cause it. The worst part was having to untell our families as only a few days before, we had begun to let everyone know that I was expecting. The next few months were pretty miserable, especially when I saw other women who were pregnant. A friend gave birth to a daughter at around the time our baby would have been due. That was quite hard as I couldn't help but wonder about what our baby might have been like. '

'When we tried again, it took quite a while to get pregnant. The first time round, I had got pregnant really quickly, but this time we were trying for nearly a year. As each month came and went, I got increasingly worried and thought that it had to be down to the earlier miscarriage. Once I did get pregnant, the doctor was fantastic. An early scan was arranged at 10 weeks to put my mind at rest. Once I saw the heart beating, I felt deep down that it would be fine. The whole pregnancy just felt different.'

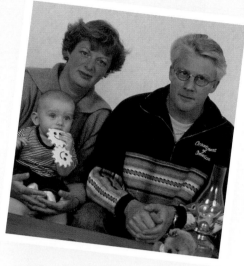

Fiona, 44 and Andrew, 50, have Archie who is now two years old.

'After Archie was born, I was keen to have another baby soon as I knew I wasn't getting any younger. When I next missed my period we were delighted. Because of my age I had an early scan just to be sure. When I set off, I was full of excitement even though Andrew couldn't be with me. As soon as they started the scan I knew something was wrong. The radiographer looked concerned and called in the doctors. They tried to break the news to me gently that there was no sign of a heartbeat. I just sobbed and couldn't really understand why as I still felt pregnant.'

'In hospital they dealt with the physical side very efficiently. I had a D and C, which left me feeling very empty, and they offered to refer me to a miscarriage clinic, but I decided not to go. The next few weeks were awful. While physically I had to cope with enormous hormonal changes, we also struggled with the most intense grief and I would cry uncontrollably for hours. For Andrew it was particularly hard as he felt there was nothing he could do – he had no role.'

'I decided not to tell people because I didn't want to be pitied or told that it was all for the best. For a while afterwards, I found it hard to see other pregnant women. It takes time to move on and I needed to work through the grief. We are ready to try again, but looking back, I wish that I had started thinking about a family sooner as I now know that being older can make a difference.'

Some possible causes of miscarriage	What it means	What you can do
Genetic	About half of all miscarriages are caused by chance genetic abnormalities in the fertilised egg. Very rarely there may be a chromosome abnormality in either the mother or the father.	There is no need to do anything. The chances of it re-occuring are slight. If you have had several miscarriages you may want to take a test for abnormalities.
Hormonal Polycystic ovary syndrome (PCOS)	This means that the ovaries are not releasing eggs regularly or at all.	Consult your doctor if you have irregular periods. Once this condition has been diagnosed you can be given drugs to correct the hormonal irregularities.
Endometriosis	This is where the tissue that lines the womb grows elsewhere in the pelvis, causing possible damage to the fallopian tubes.	Consult your doctor if you have very heavy and painful periods. Tests can be done, followed by surgery on the tubes if necessary.
Infections Fever	A fever over 39°C (100F) can cause miscarriage.	If you develop a fever when pregnant, take steps to reduce it. for example by sponging down with tepid water. Consult your doctor or midwife especially if you have been in contact with rubella or chickenpox.
Vaginal infections	Some infections can cause miscarriage, although most are easily treatable.	If you get a stinging or burning sensation when urinating or an unusual discharge seek treatment immediately.
Chlamydia (see also p.55)	Chlamydia can be sexually-transmitted or caught from cattle or sheep during lambing or calving.	Both the mother and her partner need to have a medical checkup and treatment if necessary to prevent reinfection. Avoid animals during lambing and calving!
Listeria (see also p.41)	Listeria is an infection found in unpasteurised cheese.	Avoid eating unpasteurised cheese if you think you are pregnant, or if you are planning to get pregnant.
Toxoplasmosis (see also p.53)	Toxoplasmosis is an infection caused by a tiny parasite that is found on contaminated food.	Cook meat thoroughly. Wash fruit and vegetables before eating. Wear gloves when gardening. Avoid changing cats' litter trays.
Smoking, alcohol and drugs	There is a 30–50% increased risk of miscarriage from active and passive smoking.	The safest advice is to give up smoking, alcohol and drugs completely or if you can't, cut down as much as possible (see page 51 for tips).
Work hazards exposure to solvents	Some chemicals such as solvents increase the risk of miscarriage.	If you think there may be risks in your work environment, it is worth checking with your health and safety representative. Avoid dangerous substances such as drugs.
Immune system problems Anti-phospholipid syndrome	Antibodies circulate in the blood and damage the placenta so that the baby dies.	If you have repeated miscarriages, you may be offered treatment to prevent this from occurring.
Maternal blood incompatibility	If a woman's blood is rhesus negative and the fetus is rhesus positive, the woman produces antibodies which attack the fetal cells. This causes a miscarriage.	An injection known as 'anti-D' is given after a miscarriage to prevent further miscarriages.
Anatomical problems Weak ('incompetent') cervix	The cervix opens too soon, leading to premature labour.	A stitch can be put into the neck of the womb until a few weeks before the baby is due to be born, so preventing the cervix from opening.
Irregular-shaped womb or fibroids in the womb	The baby can't grow because there isn't enough room in the womb.	Visit your doctor if you have repeated miscarriages or difficulties in conceiving.

Reducing the risks

THERE IS NO SUCH THING AS A GUARANTEED PREGNANCY. BUT THERE ARE A FEW THINGS THAT WOMEN AND INDEED THEIR PARTNERS CAN DO TO TIP THE ODDS IN FAVOUR OF A HEALTHY PREGNANCY.

Before pregnancy

You can cut down on the risk of miscarriage if you are both in good shape before getting pregnant. As half the genetic information comes from men's sperm, these need to be in good condition too! Aim to take care of yourselves for at least three months before you plan to start a family.

And also for women......

Check your immunity to childhood diseases If necessary, get checked for any infections such as chlamydia.

In the early days of a pregnancy

Once you know that you are pregnant, try and take a little bit more care of yourself. Hard as it may seem, especially if you have already experienced a miscarriage, the best advice is to try not to worry.

Rest and take it easy

Give your body the chance to rest and relax. This is so that all the body's energies can focus on the developing baby. When you stop moving around and rest your womb is also quiet and relaxed, which improves the blood flow to the placenta and the baby.

Follow the advice of your GP, midwife or consultant

If you have already had a miscarriage or stillbirth, you may have been given some advice. Make sure that you follow this carefully as it will have been tailored to your needs.

Avoid stress

Stress can have an effect on your body. Look for ways of avoiding stressful situations if possible. Try to avoid worrying about the pregnancy too although this may be easier said than done. Meet up with friends, go to the cinema or enjoy an evening in with a favourite video.

Give up smoking and alcohol

Alcohol and smoking are both poisons for the body. If you have not stopped, you should straight away. Smoking increases the risk of miscarriage by as much as 50%.

Avoid coffee and caffeine drinks

Caffeine in coffee and some energy drinks can be harmful. Drink no more than three cups per day or switch to decaffeinated.

TOGETHER ...

Stop or at least cut back on smoking

Cut down on alcohol

Get in shape and eat well

Check with your GP whether any prescribed medicines might affect your fertility

Talk to your GP if either of you have any inherited genetic conditions in your family e.g. sickle cell anaemia

Take folic acid

Folic acid is a vital vitamin for the developing baby. Take the recommended dose of 400 mcg while you are trying for a baby and also for the first 12 weeks of the pregnancy.

Eat well and avoid constipation

It is a good idea to avoid getting constipated because straining to go to the toilet might affect a pregnancy that is already at risk of miscarriage. Eating five portions of fruit and vegetables a day should help to keep the bowels regular.

Do not use recreational or street drugs

The effects of some drugs are simply not known although cannabis especially with tobacco is linked to miscarriages (see p.48).

Having sex

Once a pregnancy is well established there is no way that having sex can affect it. You should use a condom if you have sex with a new partner as a precaution against any possible infections. It may be worth avoiding using sex toys to reduce the risk of infection.

If you have had several miscarriages, your doctor may advise against having sex until after the twelfth or fourteenth week.

Avoid strenuous exercise

Gentle exercise is generally good for you, but you should avoid taking up any new sports that are strenuous, as your body will not be used to them. If you have already had a miscarriage, get some advice before carrying on with very physical sports or ones where there is a high risk of falling such as horse-riding.

Causes of INFERTILITY

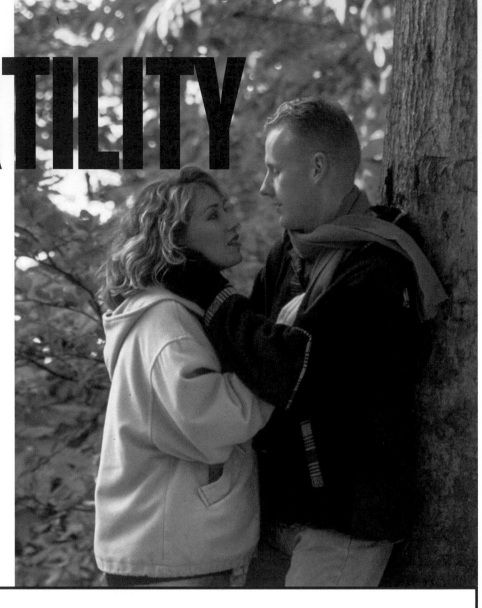

WHEN YOU DON'T GET PREGNANT

If you have decided you want a baby then not getting pregnant can be devastating. But it is surprisingly common. One in seven couples are affected by infertility at some point in their lives, but the good news is that even those who have not conceived for three years, the likelihood of getting pregnant in the end is 25%.

Fertility treatment has made great progress and there are now many options available. We answer some common questions.

WHY CAN'T I GET PREGNANT?

It is an emotional thing when you don't get pregnant. Very often people blame themselves and think it is their fault. Women can feel guilty and think, 'I'm not a proper woman if I can't have a baby'. For men it can be particularly hard, especially if the reason for the infertility is because of them – a low sperm count for example. Often couples find it difficult to admit that there is a problem and don't go for treatment. But there can be lots of reasons for infertility, many of which can be treated with great success.

Causes of infertility in women

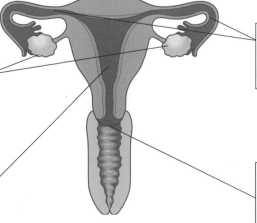

Ovaries
- May not be producing eggs. This could be for a number of reasons for example polycystic ovary syndrome (PCOS).
- The eggs may not be released.
- There may be damage from 'endometriosis' or cysts.

Fallopian tubes
- May be blocked because of a previous infection or operations, so that the sperm cannot get through to meet the egg.

Womb/uterus
- May be an abnormal shape, so the egg cannot implant itself and grow.
- May contain fibroids or polyps, (growths inside the womb), which prevent the egg from attaching itself.

Cervix
- May be partly opened so that infection gets in and damages the embryo.
- May produce hostile mucus that kills the sperm as they try to swim through to fertilise the egg.

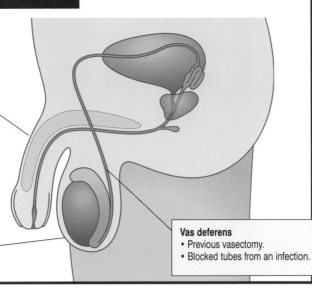

Causes of infertility in men

Penis
• Problems with ejaculation, or impotence.

Testes
• Low sperm count, which may be the result of hormonal problems of previous illnesses such as mumps, or a number of other reasons like smoking and too much heat.
• Poor quality sperm, which are not strong enough to swim up into the woman's fallopian tubes.
• Enlarged veins within the testes, called 'varicocoele', which prevent the sperm from passing through.

Vas deferens
• Previous vasectomy.
• Blocked tubes from an infection.

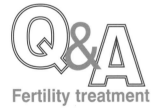

But very often there is no particular reason why a couple may be having difficulty in conceiving. It could be due to stress or just a question of time. When all the investigations have been done and there is nothing obviously wrong physically with either the man or the woman, it is called 'unexplained infertility'.

WHEN SHOULD WE GO FOR HELP?

This depends on how you feel, but 85% of couples will normally conceive after one year, it is a good idea to seek help after twelve months. There may be a reason why you are not conceiving which can be treated. Visit your GP or your local family planning clinic.

SO WHAT HAPPENS IF YOU DECIDE TO GO FOR TREATMENT?

First of all your GP or family planning nurse will want to find out if there is any reason why you aren't getting pregnant. They will check whether you have had any previous illnesses or operations, whether either of you have any problems, such as irregular periods for the woman, and how often and at what time of the month you have sex. The questions can be embarrassing, but it is essential to check that there isn't a simple explanation for the problem. Some people may just not be having sex at the most fertile time of the woman's cycle.

The next step is some simple tests. For the woman there are blood and urine tests to check that ovulation has taken place. For men there is a semen analysis to check the quality, quantity and mobility of sperm. The family planning clinic can also do a postcoital check, where 12 hours after making love the mucus in the woman's vagina is checked for live healthy sperm.

Other investigations are ultrasound and laparoscopy – a procedure where a small camera is used to see what is going on inside your body. Finally, if there is still no sign of a pregnancy, the couple may then want to consider fertility treatment, or 'assisted conception'.

Q&A
Fertility treatment

Q We have found out that the reason I'm not getting pregnant is because my partner's sperm count is low. Now he has completely gone off sex. Is this normal?
A It is not unusual for couples to find baby making stressful. Making love can become clinical and your partner may feel he is a failure because he can't get you pregnant. It might be a good idea to take a break from baby making and to spend time doing things together that you both enjoy, to remind you why you wanted to be together in the first place.

Q I've read that if you have IVF you are more likely to have twins or triplets. Is this true?
A IVF involves replacing fertilised embryos into the womb. Because the treatment involved in creating live embryos is long and hard for the couple, and unfortunately there is a risk that the embryos may still die once implanted, the doctors try to increase the chances of a pregnancy by implanting several embryos at the same time. The authorities recommend that only two embryos are implanted, but in some circumstances they may allow three. This obviously increases the chances of having a multiple birth. After discussion with the doctor you will be given the choice of how many embryos are reimplanted, up to the maximum of three.

Q My partner was married before and had 3 children and then a vasectomy. Now we are together we want to have a baby of our own. What choices do we have?
A Has your partner had his vasectomy reversed? If not then you might want to consider this as a first step. It is a delicate operation, which involves unblocking the tube which carries the sperm from the testicles to the penis. He would have to have an anaesthetic and would need to stay in hospital for a day or so, but there is a 30–70% chance that he would then produce sperm as normal. Your second option is to consider using a sperm donor (DI or donor insemination). This would involve using sperm that was not your partner's to make you pregnant. You might want to discuss this option very carefully with your partner before taking it because he would not be the natural father of the baby.

Q After we'd been trying for a baby for eighteen months I went to the doctor. He couldn't find anything wrong with me and says he needs to see my husband. But he refuses to go.
A A good start may be to explain to your husband that in the first instance, the doctor will probably just want to check out his overall health. This does not mean giving a semen sample there and then as this is usually carried out at assisted conception clinics. In some cases, men can make quite small changes to their lifestyles and improve their sperm count. If your husband still refuses, you may need to talk about your feelings as in the long term his refusal is likely to create tension and resentment in your relationship.

What are the options for fertility treatment?

Our quick guide gives you a summary of information, though your assisted conception unit or fertility clinic will be able to provide you with information to meet your own needs.

For Women

Treatment	How it works	What it means for you
Fertility pills 'Clomiphene'	Tablets for 5 days in each monthly cycle to make the ovaries produce eggs regularly.	This treatment has a 65% success rate if the periods are restored.
HMG injections	Injections from the beginning of the cycle until just before ovulation to improve egg production. This treatment is used as part of IVF.	Has to be carefully monitored by your doctor. There is a higher risk of twins or triplets.
Pump therapy	Giving hormones through a pump worn on the arm to make the ovaries produce eggs.	This is a good way to give hormones, because the pump mimics the body.
Nasal spray 'Buselin'	A spray into the nose every 4 hours. This slows down the ovaries so they respond better to HMG injections.	Particularly good for treating polycystic ovaries in preparation for IVF.
Treatment for endometriosis	This is done using drugs or microsurgery.	The success rate is variable so the surgery is only recommended when the condition is severe.
Tubal surgery	This involves operating on blocked or scarred fallopian tubes to open them up.	Although the results won't be immediate, there is a 60% chance of conception after the operation, depending on the nature and extent of the tubal damage.
Operating on the uterus (womb)	This can be a major operation to remove fibroids or open up the cavity in the uterus.	There is a 65% to 75% chance of getting pregnant after successful surgery on the womb.

For Men

Treatment	How it works	What it means for you
Fertility drugs 'Mesterolone' and 'gonadotrophin' to improve sperm count	Tablets or injections to increase the activity of the testes.	Unfortunately the evidence suggests that drug treatment for men is not very effective.
Varicocele treatment	This is a short operation where the blocked vein in the testicle is tied off or removed with a chemical injection.	This is a short and painless operation so is worth trying as some men have an improved sperm count afterwards.
Reversing a vasectomy	A delicate operation where the tiny narrow tube from the testes to the penis is unblocked.	The success rate varies from 35% to 71%.

Assisted conception

Treatment	How it works	What it means for you
IUI (Intrauterine insemination)	Specially selected and washed sperm are placed into the partner's womb using fine plastic tubing. The woman usually takes fertility drugs beforehand.	This method can be successful when there are problems with the cervix or the man's sperm quality.
DI (Donor insemination)	This is when sperm from a donor is put into a woman's vagina or womb. It is offered to couples if the man has very few sperm, or has had a vasectomy, or carries an inherited disease.	Although the chances of a pregnancy are high, this needs careful thinking about beforehand, because the woman's partner will not be the baby's natural father.
IVF ('in vitro fertilisation' or test tube babies)	This is where an egg is taken from the woman, fertilised with her partner's sperm in a test tube and replanted into her womb.	This is now a widely used procedure and has a one in five chance of success each time it is tried. However it can be a lengthy and traumatic process for the couple.
GIFT (gamete intrafallopian transfer)	Newer than IVF, this treatment involves taking eggs from the ovaries, mixing them with the partner's sperm and immediately replacing them into the fallopian tubes before fertilisation has taken place.	This is an alternative to IVF, which is sometimes used when there is no obvious reason for the infertility.
ICSI (intracytoplasmic sperm injection)	A relatively new treatment, this is where an individual's sperm, which has been specially prepared, is injected directly into the partner's egg. It is done to bypass any barriers to conception, such as blocked tubes.	This treatment has worked when IVF has failed and when the man has a low sperm count. It offers another chance to couples who have been through all the other treatments.

It's all in the genes

Blue eyes, brown eyes. Tall or short. It's all a question of what's in your genes. We look at the part genetics plays in the make up of your baby.

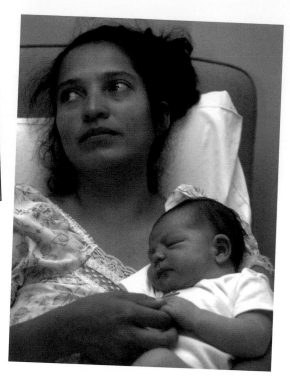

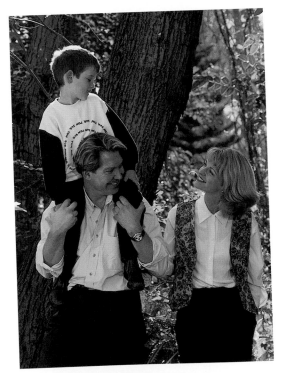

Most people look like their natural parents in some way. As well as appearance, the chances are that they may also have one or two medical conditions that run in the family such as short sightedness, asthma or hayfever. The reason behind all of this is our genes and scientists today are learning about each and every part of the genetic code that makes us the people we are.

Every cell in our body (with the exception of the sperm and ovum) contains 46 chromosomes. These are grouped in pairs, making 23 pairs. The chromosomes act like a library of information. The chromosomes are in turn made up of long threads of a chemical that has become known as DNA (deoxyribonucleic acid). Each thread has segments called genes. It is thought that humans have around 50,000 genes. It is the genes that determine our physical characteristics such as our skin colour, height and shape of our faces, plus perhaps having some influence on our personalities, intelligence and physical talents.

Genes are also linked to our health as it is becoming clear that faulty genes can cause diseases and some genes may pre-dispose us to some conditions.

Your baby's unique inheritance

Your baby will get half of their chromosomes and genetic information from you and the other half from your partner. This is because while normal human cells have 46 chromosomes, the sperm and the egg only have 23 each. The make up of the 23 chromosomes in the man's sperm and the woman's egg is a random selection and this is why children with the same parents are not the same. At the moment of conception the sperm fuses with the egg and the chromosomes pair off. The genetic lottery has then begun. Everyone, with the exception of identical twins, has their own unique DNA make-up. Identical twins have the same DNA make up because shortly after conception, the fertilised egg splits into two.

Problems with DNA

Like most processes, conception and the copying of genes is not completely problem free. Sometimes chromosomes are damaged or the wrong number are produced. The risk of this happening increases with age as the genetic information in a woman's eggs will be the same age as her. When this happens, a woman may have a miscarriage or a child may be born with some kind of developmental delay. This is one reason why many fertility experts are keen for women who are thinking about starting a family to begin earlier rather than later.

As well as damaged or extra chromosomes, some genes that we inherit are faulty. In many cases, this has no effect on us at all as the genes are 'switched off'. Unfortunately, combined with our partner's genetic information, they can sometimes be switched back on again. This is why certain conditions such as colour blindness, cystic fibrosis and sickle cell anaemia can jump generations. If all this sounds alarming, it is worth remembering that nature tends to get it right more often than wrong and so genetic conditions are reasonably rare.

Miscarriages

A high percentage of miscarriages will be caused because nature's lottery has not worked out. The genetic information in the developing embryo can be faulty and this causes the pregnancy to stop.

Genetic
COUNSELLING
Do we need it?

While nature plays a sort of lottery, sometimes the odds of having a baby with a serious hereditary illness can be predicted. For couples worried about passing on a life-threatening disease or serious birth defect, it is now possible to find out the actual risks by going through genetic counselling.

What does genetic counselling do?

The aim of genetic counselling is to provide couples with information and support so they can make informed choices. Genetic counsellors do not push couples in any particular direction, so the couples decisions are very much their own and depend on the disease and their own feelings. In some cases, couples will decide to let nature take its course, others may ask for IVF treatment, while others may decide to use donor sperm or eggs.

How does genetic counselling work?

Genetic counselling is carried out by specialist counsellors who have a nursing or medical background. It is a very sensitive area so counsellors are chosen very carefully. Couples may be asked about their family history as well as for a blood test or a swab. The information allows the counsellor to calculate the risk of disease being passed on to a child. Alongside this information, couples are then talked through their own feelings about the risk and about the possible options that may be available.

Why do people go for genetic counselling?

Genetic counselling is not about creating designer babies. Couples tend to seek genetic counselling because they want to avoid having a baby with a serious disease or wish to understand the risk of this happening. They may already have a baby with a disorder, know that they are a carrier or have a close member of their family who has a life threatening disease.

Name of disease	Effects	Inheritance pattern	Incidence	What you can do
Sickle cell anemia	Serious and painful blood disorder.	Both parents must pass on a copy of this gene.	Found mainly in the UK among people of African and Caribbean descent. Estimated 1 in 10–40 people will carry the gene.	Consider seeking advice if you are both from this group and if either of you have close relatives with this illness.
Tay Sachs	Life threatening progressive illness.	Both parents must pass on a copy of this gene.	Found mainly in the UK amongst Askhenazi Jews. Estimated 1 in 25 will carry the gene.	Consider seeking advice if you are both from this group and if either of you have close relatives with this illness.
Cystic fibrosis	Life threatening progressive illness.	Both parents must pass on a copy of this gene.	Found mainly amongst people of white Western European descent. Estimated 1 in 25 will carry the gene.	Consider seeking advice if you are both from this group and if either of you have close relatives with this illness.
Thalassaemia	Life threatening blood disorder.	Both parents must pass on a copy of this gene.	Found mainly in the UK among people from Mediterranean, Middle Eastern or Asiandescent.	Consider seeking advice if you are both from this group and if either of you have close relatives with this illness.

The decision on whether to go for genetic counselling is a difficult choice for many couples. Perhaps both partners feel differently about the decision? Here we answer some of the common concerns surrounding this topic.

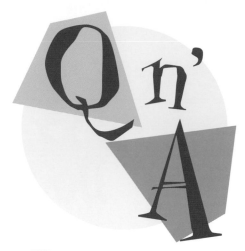

We answer some of the common concerns on genetic counselling

Q How do we get help?

A First of all, it is important not to panic and to seek the support and advice of your family doctor. She will talk through your concerns with you and will, if required, refer you for genetic counselling. It may be that while there is a member of your family with a disease, there is no risk of this being passed on.

Q I am thirty-six years old and worried about my chance of having a baby with Down's syndrome.

A The risk of having a child with Down's syndrome does increase dramatically with a woman's age. Talk through the statistics and risks with your doctor and also your partner. Tests can be carried out in pregnancy to detect babies who have chromosomal disorders. While some couples decide not to continue with such pregnancies, others do and go on to have and love their children.

Q There is a history of mental illness in my family. I am worried about passing this on.

A It is important that you start by going to your doctor and talking through your concerns. Not all types of mental illness are hereditary and while this was very much a taboo subject a few years ago, attitudes and treatment are changing. You will need to find out as much as you can about your family history, both medical and social. In some cases, people were wrongly diagnosed as having mental illnesses when in fact they had underlying emotional difficulties or medical illnesses.

Q My husband is desperate for a boy. Will we be able to ask for treatment to select only male embryos?

A Genetics is a very sensitive topic and sex selection is very carefully regulated. At present, doctors will only carry out treatment to select the sex of a baby if there is a significant medical reason for doing so. You can however try tipping the odds in your favour through some DIY techniques (see p.19), but note that these are not guaranteed.

Q I am heavily overweight and have dieted all my life. Will I be at risk of having children who are overweight?

A While it is thought that there may be some genetic link to obesity, the food that you eat and your activity level play a more important role. Put simply, your activity level must balance with the calories that you are taking in. Begin by seeking advice and support about your own diet and attitudes towards food. You can make an appointment with your family doctor, practice nurse or consider joining a reputable slimming club. This will help you to make sure that you pass on good eating habits and healthy attitudes towards food to your children.

SHOULD WE GO FOR GENETIC COUNSELLING?

Overall very few couples will need genetic counselling, but it is advisable to talk to your doctor before you get pregnant if you have any concerns.

- **Does either of your parents or close relatives have an inherited disease or birth defect?**

- **Have either of you already had a child with a birth defect or genetic disorder?**

- **Have you had two or more miscarriages?**

- **Are you closely related e.g. first cousins or have a closely related family tree?**

- **You are aware that you may at risk because of your shared racial or ethnic descent (see table on p.77)**

If you're a man then you might not have thought about how a woman's body works or pregnancy since school days.

Here we explain a bit more about getting pregnant, the pregnancy itself and how you might be feeling.

Do you know much about sperm? Test your knowledge with our fun quiz on page 84. Depending on how much you know or how well you do in the quiz, you might want to read our tips on how to make your sperm count!

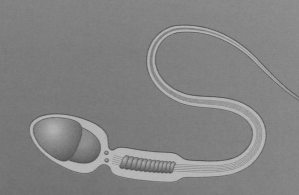

82–84
pages

Have you ever thought "I don't know what my partner's thinking or how to deal with her"? Maybe you're not the only one – we answer some of the common questions men ask about trying for a baby.

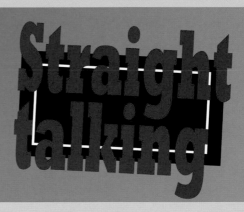

Straight talking

85
page

Back to basics

If your knowledge of conception is rusty or you have never really mastered 'women's stuff', it's worth getting to grips with it. A bit of knowledge can make quite a difference.

The process

When men ejaculate or 'come' into a woman's vagina, millions of sperm contained in the semen begin to travel up to the vagina. Some go into a woman's womb and then onto the fallopian tubes. Very few make it but once there, one sperm needs to meet up with an egg for conception to take place. Once conception takes place the fertilised egg travels down the fallopian tubes and attaches itself to the side of the womb where a special lining has been prepared. Here it grows and develops for the next nine months.

Women are not fertile all the time

A woman is not fertile all the time. Her body releases an egg each month from one of her ovaries. If the egg is not fertilised, it is passed out through the vagina along with the special lining that the womb prepared. This is the monthly bleed or period that a woman has. The whole process of producing an egg is controlled by a woman's hormones. It is these hormones that can contribute towards women's mood swings.

When is the best time?

There are certain days each month where you should aim to have sex if you are trying for a baby. This is when your partner's body is releasing an egg. This is called ovulation. If you have sex just before or during ovulation, there is a better chance of fertilisation taking place.

How long does it take?

Conception, depends on many factors including the health of you and your partner, timing of sex and of course luck. Anything up to one year is quite normal, although for some couples it does not take long and they conceive in the first month. If nothing has happened after about a year or before if it is getting stressful, you should consider visiting your doctor together.

How do you find out?

When women are pregnant, they usually stop having periods. There are also other signs such as feeling sick, feeling very tired and having sore breasts. A pregnancy test that can be done either in a clinic or at home will give a definite result.

What happens next?

Once your partner knows she is pregnant, she can make an appointment to see the doctor. It is a good idea to go along too so that you can support her and learn more about what will happen in the next few months. She will be given details of the antenatal care and appointments that she should attend.

Can anything go wrong?

Nature is not perfect and quite often pregnancies do stop. This leads to a miscarriage where a woman bleeds as the material from the pregnancy is disposed of. While miscarriages are common, emotionally they are very painful both for women and men.

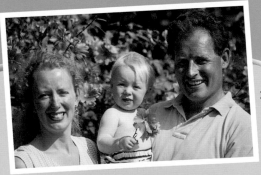

Mike 34 and Emily 31 have Grace 8 months.

Mike was happy to start a family, but was surprised to find that it doesn't always happen straight away.

'I suppose I had always been brought up to believe that women's things were definitely best left to women. Emily had never been one to talk about her periods and so most of the time I can honestly say I didn't really know much about that side at all. We started trying for a baby after our summer holiday. I didn't think too much about it. I just thought you get on with it and boom, you would have a baby! I've learnt a lot since then though.

After three months, Emily was beginning to get a bit anxious and I was a bit surprised that we hadn't done it. It's funny because although I have got some good mates and they had kids, no one really talks about the getting pregnant side of things. We waited for another couple of months and then we went to see the doctor. By this time, it had got a bit stressful for both of us. I was starting to think that maybe it was me. I wasn't sure at first if I wanted to go and tell the doctor anything, but Emily insisted.

The doctor was fine and it made me realise that many couples have to get a bit of advice. She was quite matter of fact which made it easier for me. She explained that it's normal for couples to take anything up to a year but did also ask us a few questions.

Basically, she said that I needed to cut down on the amount I was drinking and should also start to wear baggy underwear. She explained that I should try to stand up more often rather than staying seated and should have cooler showers. She also went through some of the basics as to when it is best to have sex. She did warn us that it might take a few more months before Emily would get pregnant as she thought that my sperm count might have been a bit on the low side. It seemed as if I had been doing all the wrong things and it takes a while for the sperm count to build up.

Looking back, going together to see the doctor was probably the best thing we could have done. Afterwards I found that it was much easier for Emily and I to talk things through and I learnt much more about her body. Two months later, Emily realised that she was pregnant.'

Have you got what it takes?

What's it like to be a father?

We ask fathers to tell us how it is.

If it's the first one, unless you have a very close friend or family member with children, it is a great shock. Everything in your life you have had some preparation for. You may take driving lessons before you are let out on your own, but this is different. With children, they just come and you have to get on with it.

It's very rewarding, but on the other hand very exhausting. It's great to see them grow, but to hold down a job and be a good dad is harder than you think. The best bits are things like taking them out on your bike.

They say that no book in the world can prepare you and they're right. It's knackering, but getting a cuddle at bed time or seeing their faces light up is amazing.

Before, I would leave work and go to the pub. Now I leave work, think about what needs doing at home and then may not go to the pub. Not going to the pub is not the thing that I thought it would be. It's daft, but playing football in the garden makes up for it.

I know other men who flatly wouldn't want another child because they think that it would interfere with their lives. But I love having them around and we are even thinking about having a third. It is tiring, but the love and things just outweigh the tiredness.

You've got to be involved from the start. That way you get to love them and really enjoy being with them. You can't just dip in and out for the best bits because in the end you lose out. I did everything. Nappy changing, bathing – the lot. My kids love me and I love them. I often wonder what I did before they came along.

Before, everyone kept telling me how awful it would be. I don't know if they were having me on. The sleepless nights, the crying and other stuff. So I was expecting it to be a lot worse than it was. We don't go out so much, but then when we do it's a bit more special.

Going for OPTIMUM PERFORMANCE

Mention the word fertility and most people immediately think about women. Fair enough as it's women who carry the baby. But fertility is not just about women. Men have an essential role to play in the creation of a healthy baby. We look at how to help you to your optimum performance.

SPERM ARE SPECIAL

You may not give a second thought to sperm, assuming that they will be there when needed. In reality sperm are special for two reasons.

1 They carry vital genetic material without which a healthy baby cannot be produced.
2 They have to be physically strong enough to survive the equivalent of swimming across the English Channel. Not surprisingly, many sperm do not make this incredible journey. It is estimated that of the 300 million sperm that may set out at ejaculation, only 50–100 will make it to the right place at the right time.

SPERM ARE LIKE TOP ATHLETES

You might imagine that every bloke produces the same quantity and quality of sperm. This is simply not true. In many ways, sperm are like top athletes and need to be provided with the best conditions in order for them to perform. Like top athletes, they too need preparation time before their big day. It takes a staggering 100 days for sperm to be ready and in this time, they need to be well looked after.

1 Poor diet, smoking and alcohol can lower their performance.
2 Stress and having sex too often can also reduce sperm count.

3 Sperm ideally like to be kept cooler than the rest of the body, which is why they are housed outside in the testes or balls. Wearing very tight clothing or sitting a lot can keep them at too high a temperature.

ARE YOU GIVING YOUR SPERM THE BEST?

Sperm that have second-rate conditions simply find it harder to perform. Fewer of them are likely to survive the journey to the top of a woman's fallopian tubes.

Simple ways to make your sperm count

What to do	Why
Cut down your alcohol intake	Even a moderate amount of alcohol reduction can make a real difference to male fertility.
Stop smoking	Smoking is a poison and does lower sperm count.
Wear baggy trousers and loose underwear	To create the best conditions for your sperm, you should keep your balls cool.
Avoid taking hot showers and sitting in baths	Exposure to heat increases the temperature of your balls.
Do not cycle or sit down for long periods	Cycling and sitting down for a long time again makes the balls too hot.
Eat five portions of fruit and vegetables a day	Vitamin C found in fresh fruit and vegetables makes an amazing difference to your sperm count.
Take some exercise	Aim to exercise for at least 20-30 minutes, three times a week. Very long periods of strenuous exercise will lower your sperm count. You may get the muscles, but you may not get the performance!
Avoid getting worked up	Stress can have a huge effect on conception. Stay cool and get help early on if you are worried.

WHAT HAPPENS IF I HAVE TO GIVE A SAMPLE?

If a couple are finding it hard to conceive, doctors routinely like to check out both partners. Normally semen samples are taken after a few days of abstinence from sex and are usually done in a clinic so that the sperm are still alive. Most men say the trickiest part is producing the actual sample. This is done in private with a few discreet magazines to stimulate the imagination and hopefully the erection.

Sperm tests check the following:

- **Concentration – how many sperm are being produced**
- **Progressive motility – how well sperm are able to swim and move**
- **Morphology – number of sperm and are they the correct shape and structure**

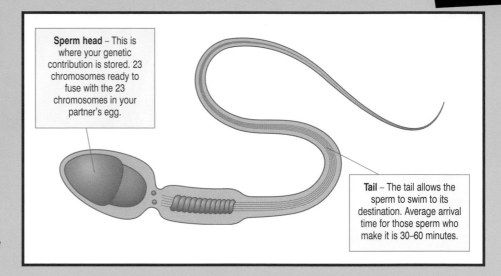

Sperm head – This is where your genetic contribution is stored. 23 chromosomes ready to fuse with the 23 chromosomes in your partner's egg.

Tail – The tail allows the sperm to swim to its destination. Average arrival time for those sperm who make it is 30–60 minutes.

THE SPERM WHO DO NOT MAKE IT TO THE TOP

Not all sperm will make it to the top of the fallopian tubes. If you are an 'average' man you are likely to produce between 100 and 300 million sperm in your semen when you ejaculate. Staggeringly, of these only 50 –100 will make the long journey.

WHY SO FEW?

1 Not all sperm will be properly formed. It is thought that many men will have up to 40% of sperm that will be abnormal.

2 Up to 20% will not be able to swim.

3 Some sperm will literally get lost on the way to the fallopian tubes.

4 Some sperm will not survive the journey.

Fact file

Sperm determine the sex of a baby.

Sperm count drops during the summer months.

Sperm counts in the male population have fallen since 1977.

HOW MUCH DO YOU KNOW ABOUT YOUR SPERM?

You are likely to take it for granted, but how much do you know about sperm?

1 How fast can sperm swim?
a) 3mm per hour
b) 3cm per hour
c) 3 metres per hour
d) 3 km per hour

2 On average, how long do sperm survive inside a woman?
a) 7–8 hours
b) 1–3 days
c) 3–5 days
d) 8–10 days

3 Alcohol plays a factor in how many cases of male infertility?
a) 10%
b) 20%
c) 30%
d) 40%

4 How long does it take the body to produce sperm ready for ejaculation?
a) 10 minutes
b) 10 hours
c) 10 days
d) 100 days

5 To improve sperm count you should ...
a) have sex twice a day
b) wear loose underwear
c) drink two pints of lager a day
d) work out each day in the gym

6 How long does it take the fittest sperm to reach the fallopian tubes?
a) 3–6 seconds
b) 3–6 minutes
c) 30–60 minutes
d) 30–60 hours

Answers

1 a Sperm have to move through a woman's cervical mucus. At the time a woman is ovulating, her mucus becomes thinner and easier for the sperm to move through.

2 c Sperm that can fertilise an egg rarely live beyond 5 days. This means that getting the timing of sex right is quite important. Ideally you should have sex around the time that a woman is ovulating.

3 d Alcohol seriously lowers sperm count even when it is quite moderate consumption. Try cutting it out or cutting down.

4 d Sperm takes nearly three months to produce from start to finish. This means that any changes made to improve the sperm count can take a while to kick in

5 b Wearing loose underwear keeps the testes cool. This improves sperm count. Having sex very frequently can lower sperm count as can drinking alcohol and exercising vigorously.

6 c It takes around 30–60 minutes, although very few sperm will make it. This is why it pays to do every thing possible to ensure sperm are the fittest they can be.

Straight talking

IT'S NOT ALWAYS EASY TO UNDERSTAND WHAT WOMEN ARE FEELING OR EVEN THINKING!

Q My partner wants me to stop smoking and even drinking. When I say that I don't see the point, she accuses me of not wanting a baby.

Smoking and drinking can both affect the quality of your sperm and so this may be the reason why she wants you to stop. Smoking after the baby is born increases the risk of cot death and of your child developing asthma. From your partner's point of view, having a healthy baby should be a priority for both of you and so this may be why she is linking your refusal to you not wanting a baby. Consider whether or not you are ready for a baby and if you are, reassure her by at least cutting down on alcohol and getting help to stop smoking (see p.64)

Q My partner seems to be completely obsessed by getting pregnant. As each month goes by, she gets more and more upset. Is this normal?

Yes! Once the decision has been made not all but most women want to conceive quickly. It is a life changing step and while a man knows when he has done his bit, women have to wait for at least a couple of weeks. The waiting is often the hardest part for women. Each month they have to wait not knowing whether or not they are pregnant. This means that when their period does come, they can be desperately disappointed as they must now wait for another whole month. Talk to your partner about when her next period is due so that you can be there, to commiserate or hopefully to celebrate with her. Also try to spend some time doing nice things together other than having sex.

Q My partner had a miscarriage a few months ago and still cries about it. I cannot seem to cheer her up.

Miscarriages can be very hard to cope with emotionally even when the physical side is over. Women can also find constant daily reminders of the child they were hoping for, as they notice prams and other pregnant women. Try listening to your partner rather than trying to cheer her up if she cries. While you may want her to snap out of it, she may still need to grieve. Knowing that you are there and trying to understand her will help enormously.

Q My wife insists on using ovulation kits. When she thinks it is the 'right time' we are supposed to get on with it, but I don't perform to order.

You are not alone. Ovulation kits can be helpful, but can also make it harder for men as the whole thing can become too clinical. Talk to your wife about how you are feeling and explore together other ways of finding out when the best time in the month to conceive is (see p.16).

Q We have been trying for a baby for nearly a year and nothing has happened. I am wondering if it could be my fault.

A First of all, it is not a good idea to start feeling guilty. Stress and anxiety can really count against conception so stop blaming yourself. Your first port of call should be to see your doctor either together or separately if you prefer. They will find out about your general health and give you some advice. In the meantime try to cut down on alcohol, wear loose fitting underwear and if you are in a job where you sit for long periods of time, aim to stand up regularly. All these simple measures can increase your sperm count, although it can take a few months for the effects to kick in.

Q My wife is worried because I work with pesticides. Can this make a difference?

Some types of work do carry health risks and can make a difference to a man's sperm. You will need to get the facts about the products that you are using. The best way is to contact the manufacturer directly or if you are employed to ask the company's health and safety officer. You could also seek advice from the Health and Safety Executive (www.hse.gov.uk)
The products will probably be safe, but you will need to follow the safety precautions to the letter. This may mean wearing protective clothing, masks and also washing hands and equipment thoroughly.

Is it time for a BABY?

Having a baby is a major step and a decision that only you can make. We look at the most common issues involved in making this decision.

THINKING ABOUT AN ADDITION?

Some men and women know they want children. That's great, but what happens if you are not sure, your partner doesn't want any children or if you don't have a partner. We look at some common dilemmas.

Q My partner keeps saying that he does not want any children. We have been together for 4 years and I am now 26 and feeling desperate. I am thinking about having 'an accident'.

A Getting pregnant and hoping that your partner will change his mind is a very high- risk strategy and one that does not often pay off. Your partner may leave you if he finds it hard to cope with the baby or simply ignore the baby and leave all the hard work to you. You could both end up feeling resentful of each other and this can put a huge strain on your relationship.

Instead try exploring why he feels as he does. Make sure that you are ready to listen and respect his views, even if they are not what you are hoping to hear. Before saying or doing anything rash, try to calmly explain how you are feeling. It could be that he is not sure about settling down yet, although he is ready to think about having children later on. Equally, he could be someone who really does not want children at all costs. If at the end of the day, he really does not want children and you know that you cannot live without having any, you will both need to make some very hard decisions about where your relationship is going.

Q We are a female gay couple wanting a baby. How should we organise this?

A As with any couple or woman wanting to have a baby, you should think carefully about how you will cope with this life change. Talk this through and think about the dynamics of your relationship and the roles that you will play. Families come in all shapes and sizes today, you should find that medical professionals will be supportive of your wishes. Do not be tempted to try and inseminate at home. There is a serious danger of picking up a sexually transmitted infection this way.

Q I am 35 years old and have just been promoted at work. The problem is that my husband is really keen to start a family. It's not that I don't want children, I just want to wait for a few more years.

A While you may be one of those lucky women who get pregnant easily in their late thirties, you do not know this for sure. A woman's fertility declines dramatically in her thirties while the risk of miscarriage and having a baby with Down's syndrome increases. This means that you will seriously need to think about what is at stake if you wait and how much of a gambler you are.

If it is your career that is the issue, look to the future. You may get further promotions so you may be facing the same dilemma later on as you are now. If you do want to start a family, you may need to start thinking about how you might juggle career and children. Plenty of women do this and have good careers. Explain to your husband how you are feeling and consider together whether his work habits could change so that he might become responsible for the eventual organisation of childcare.

Q I am a single woman with no boyfriend or partner in sight. I am now nearly 40 and know that time is running out for me.

A Bringing up a baby as a lone parent is not impossible and many women do manage, but it is very tiring, demanding and even lonely at times. You will need to think through the financial consequences of having a baby alone and how you will cope with childcare arrangements if you are working. As well as thinking about the practical demands of being a lone parent, you should also ask yourself why you want a baby and whether you will use the child as an emotional crutch. While it is normal to love a baby and be loved in return, babies cannot be expected to fill in for an absent partner or husband.

If you make the decision to go ahead, you need to get pregnant safely. This means resisting the temptation to have a one night stand or use a friend's sperm. To do so may put you at risk of getting a sexually transmitted infection and in the case of using sperm from someone you know, there may be all kinds of emotional complications later on. This means that you need to get some medical advice and help. Visit your doctor or local family planning clinic and explain your situation. They should help you to access donated sperm, although there may be a fee for this.

Q I already have a teenage daughter by my first marriage. My new partner is really keen for us to have a baby together, but I am not sure how my daughter will react.

A First of all, ask yourself if you are using your teenage daughter as an excuse. Is it that deep down you do not want a baby or that you are unsure about how this relationship is going? If this is not the case, then think about your relationship with your daughter. Most teenagers, after the initial surprise, enjoy having a baby in the family, providing that they do not feel dislodged by the newcomer. Consider if she needs more attention and reassurances from you and your new partner.

Finally, this is one decision that you and your partner must take together. You should both be honest and consider how you will feel in a few years' time if you decide not to have a baby.

Career or baby?

Can women have it both ways?

YEARS AGO, WOMEN HAD LITTLE OPTION BUT TO STAY AT HOME WHEN THEIR CHILDREN WERE SMALL. NOWADAYS, THERE ARE MORE OPTIONS FOR WOMEN TO RETURN TO WORK. WE TALK TO TWO WOMEN ABOUT THE CHOICES THEY MADE.

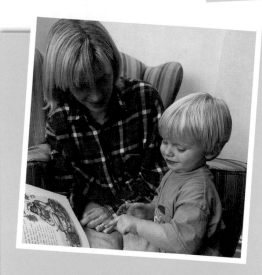

Gail (27), Paul (30) with Toby (2)

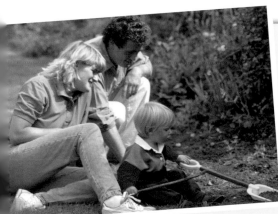

Mandy (32), Dave (35) and Josh aged 2 years

'I knew that I wanted to continue with my job after Josh was born. Not only did I enjoy my work, but, to be honest, it would have been very hard going financially. After Josh was born, I fell deeply in love with him. Nothing prepares you for this and it was quite a shock to find myself thinking about staying at home with him. We found a childminder close to where we live and from five months old, I used to leave him for the odd morning so that he and I got in the habit of being apart. The first time I left him was really hard, but when I picked him up he was fine and I felt that it had gone well. When I started back at work, I was a bit worried that I would feel 'out of it' but everyone was pleased to see me back and by the end of morning, it felt like I had not been away. I hardly thought about Josh at all, although at the end of the day I was desperate to pick up. Josh is now two years old and it is working out really well, although it is tiring to come home from work and then find the energy to play and spend time with him. Dave and I try and work out our holidays so that we can have some time together with him, but also so that we have the odd day off with him by ourselves.

There have been times when I have felt guilty about being a working mother. I know that I am not alone though because other working mothers say the same thing. The guilt can come from the odd comment that people make, but the worst guilt comes from inside me and you have to learn to manage this. You also need to make sure that you are 100% happy with the person who is looking after your child, so that you can get along in the day with your job without worrying.'

'We decided to start a family earlier rather than later. Someone I knew at work had left it quite late and then not managed to conceive and so I think that this shaped my decision to get on with it rather than leave it until later. We also felt it would be easier to survive without money, if we hadn't actually got used to having any in the first place. I did enjoy my job, but I also knew that I wanted to be at home for the baby. It was hard at first being at home especially during the first six or seven months. I realised that I didn't really know anybody with babies and of course most of my friends were at work. Things have changed a lot now because I have got my own circle of friends and I have much more of a pattern to the week.

The other thing about being at home is that you don't get much time for yourself. At work, I was used to having a lunch hour or a few minutes break, but at home, you are on the go nearly all the time. It's quite hard sometimes to feel that you have achieved anything. In my old job, I could see what I had done especially when a project was finished, but being at home you don't get that same sense of achievement. Hanging out the washing or reading the paper for ten minutes isn't something to feel good about and you can get to feel quite down unless you do something for yourself each week. In my case, I have started to study again as I have had a chance to think about what I really want to do once I go back to work. It's a bit like having an early career break. Money is tight, though, and we do watch what we spend, although when we go out, it's more of a treat than before. I know that not having much to spend won't last forever and being with Toby is more important for me.'

Finding out about
CHILDCARE

THE KEY TO RETURNING TO WORK IS TO FIND GOOD AND AFFORDABLE CHILDCARE. IT IS A GOOD IDEA TO FIND OUT ABOUT CHILDCARE IN YOUR AREA BEFORE THE BIRTH OF YOUR CHILD SO THAT YOU CAN WORK OUT THE COSTS AND ALSO CHECK OUT THE AVAILABILITY.

WHERE TO FIND OUT ABOUT CHILDCARE

Every local authority has been asked by the government to provide information about childcare. To find out about the Children's Information Service in your local area, phone 0800 096 02 96 or log on to www.childcarelink.gov.uk

CHILDMINDERS, NANNIES AND AU PAIRS

Childminders	Look after babies and children in their own homes. Can offer full and part time places. Many children carry on going to their childminder after school. Their practice and homes are inspected.	Children's information service Local newspaper Word of mouth
Nannies	Care for babies and children in your own home. Can live in with you. Some nannies are happy to be shared with another family. As they are not inspected or registered, it is a good idea only to use qualified nannies.	Nanny agencies Put in an advert in local newspaper or national magazine such as *The Lady* or *Nursery World*
Au pair	Care for children alongside the parents or for very short periods. Au pairs are not meant to have sole responsibility for children as they are often not trained, registered or inspected.	Nanny agency Local newspaper

NURSERIES AND PRE-SCHOOLS
ALL NURSERIES AND PRE-SCHOOLS ARE REGISTERED AND INSPECTED

Day care nurseries	Most day care nurseries take babies and also open long hours so that parents can go on to work.	Children's information service Local newspaper Word of mouth
Workplace nurseries	As above, but are based in an employer's workplace or nearby.	Children's information service Human resources or personnel department
Nursery schools	Usually take children from two years upwards and often only in term times.	Children's information service Local newspaper Word of mouth
Pre-schools	Usually offer sessional care for children over two years e.g. mornings or afternoons. Are usually not open for long hours.	Children's information service Local newspaper Word of mouth

What are your rights?

Maternity leave

You are entitled to 26 weeks maternity leave regardless of how long you have worked for your employer. The earliest you can take this maternity leave is 11 weeks before the baby is due. Depending on how long you have worked with your employer you may be entitled to some paid leave. When you return to work, your employer must give you back your old job/similar job on the same terms and conditions.

Additional maternity leave

If by the fifteenth week before your baby is due, you have been employed for 26 continuous weeks, you are entitled to take additional maternity leave. This can last a further 26 weeks from the date the ordinary maternity leave finishes. This will not be paid leave. When you return to work, your employer must find you a job which has the same status and conditions as your old job.

Paternity leave

Fathers can take one or two weeks off work any time within the 56-week period of the expected date of birth. Fathers have to have worked for at least 26 weeks and can claim a paternity leave payment.

Time off for dependents

Your employer has to give you time off if you have a family emergency such as illness of a child or childcare problem. This is usually unpaid leave.

Returning to work after leave

You must give your employer 28 days notice of your intention to return to work after either type of leave.

Parental leave

If you have worked for more than one year with an employer, either you or your partner can apply for parental leave. This is unpaid leave and allows each of you to have three months for each child. You have to show that this will be used for the purpose of caring for a child of under five years unless the child has a disability.

Flexible working

All employers now have to consider requests from men and women if they wish to change their hours because they have young children under five years old. This can also mean that you can ask to work part time rather than full time. You must apply for flexible working in writing and you must have been in continuous employment for a minimum of 26 weeks.

Money Clinic

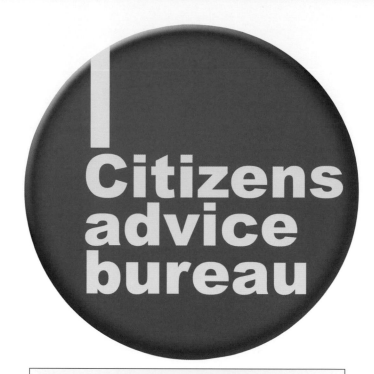

Citizens advice bureau

WITH NEWSPAPERS RUNNING HEADLINES SUGGESTING THAT HAVING CHILDREN CAN COST A FORTUNE, IT'S NOT SURPRISING THAT MANY PEOPLE WORRY ABOUT WHETHER THEY CAN AFFORD A BABY.

Citizens Advice Bureau (CAB) give impartial and confidential advice on a wide range of topics. You can find information about the benefit system, your employment rights and also advice if you are in debt or have difficulties with shops and services. Information is free. To find out about your nearest CAB, look in your local telephone directory or go to www.adviceguide.org.uk

HOW EXPENSIVE IS IT?

It is worth remembering that babies are not in themselves expensive. They do not come into the world demanding designer cots, clothes or toys. Most parents find that it is only in children's teenage years that the food and clothing becomes a real expense. The chief expense is actually the cost of childcare or if you decide not to return to work, the loss of a regular income. This is the figure that usually makes headline news and can cause people to panic . The reality is that thousands of parents each year are able to manage financially. So how do they do it?

GETTING USED TO HAVING LESS MONEY

It's an old saying that you spend up to what you earn. Most couples find that while money is tight after having children, they are able to adjust to having less money. Some couples even wonder what they were spending it on before! If you are unsure about whether or not you can cope, one suggestion is to keep a money diary for a month. This will show you exactly where your money is going. Takeaway foods, drinks, evenings out and clothes are often some of the main culprits. The question at the end of the month to consider is if you are ready to lower your standard and cost of living in order to have a baby.

SAVING AND PAYING OFF DEBTS

Once you know where your money is going, ideally you should start to save. Some couples open separate savings accounts to make sure they don't spend it. Having your own 'baby fund' can be a great incentive.

If you have debts, you should look at ways of reducing them. Paying off debts can in the longer term save money even if you cannot pay them off in full. Consider going to seek free professional help at your local Citizens Advice Bureau or contacting an independent financial advisor.

DON'T WORRY ABOUT PROVIDING PERFECTION

There is a lot of pressure when having a baby to buy expensive equipment or to feel that your home has to be perfect. The reality is that babies and young children simply do not care. A battered kitchen or old carpet in the lounge makes absolutely no difference to their happiness or your ability to be a good parent. Remembering this can save you thousands of pounds. The only baby equipment that should be bought new are safety items such as car seats. Everything else can be second hand, although you would want to check it is in good condition.

GETTING FINANCIAL HELP

There are a number of benefits and tax credits that all families can claim even those who are on higher incomes. If you are on a low income, you may also receive other financial help. To find out more, you should visit your local social security office or local branch of the Citizens Advice Bureau. You can find out the telephone numbers or addresses by looking in a phone book.

Tips for keeping financial control

- Get a hold on your spending. Keep within your income.
- Work out where the money 'black hole' is by keeping a diary.
- Try and get into the habit of saving regularly.
- Before taking on new financial commitments, think about whether they are really needed.
- Get advice and help if you are in debt.

Getting the most from your
health service

MANY PEOPLE DO NOT FEEL COMFORTABLE GOING TO THEIR DOCTOR OR GOING ALONG FOR AN APPOINTMENT AT THE HOSPITAL. WE LOOK AT WAYS WHICH WILL HELP YOU TO GET THE MOST OUT OF YOUR HEALTH SERVICE.

Visiting your doctor

Your doctor is likely to be your first port of call if you are either having difficulties in getting pregnant or are now pregnant. Unfortunately, most of us will have doctors who are quite busy and this can mean that we don't get the best out of our visits. So how can we get the most of our visit?

First of all, **be clear in your own mind** why you are going. Most doctors' appointments are for less than ten minutes so try not to waste time with the things that are not that important to you.

Next, if you are going for help because you are finding it hard to get pregnant, **be ready to talk** about your menstrual cycle and the times when you have sex in the month. Think about this information before you go in and do not be embarrassed about it. If you are pregnant, your doctor will need to know when your last period was and also may ask about your partner's medical history if you know it.

Be honest with yourself. Doctors are not mind readers and so can only go on the information you give them. If you are not honest, they will find it much harder to treat you and to give you good advice. Think about how much you really are smoking or how often you really do take exercise. Doctors these days are used to all kinds of lifestyles and goings on.

Finally, don't be afraid to **ask questions** or to tell your doctor that you do not understand something. If you find this difficult to do, make sure that you bring along your partner, a friend or a relative who can do this for you. This can be very useful because many of us forget exactly what we're told by the doctor.

Focus on midwives

Your midwife, who more than likely will be a woman, will be a key person during pregnancy. Midwives specialise in the routine care of pregnant women and the delivery of babies. They will check on your health as well as the health of your baby and you are likely to see your GP only if there is medical problem that they cannot deal with. Most women find their midwives extremely helpful and supportive and they usually have much more time than doctors. This means it can be easier to discuss emotions and feelings with them.

First visit

On your first visit, you will be able to discuss any concerns or issues that you have and also find out about how you are going to be looked after and what choices are available. For example you may want to talk about having a home birth or be cared for by the same midwife throughout the pregnancy.

Your midwife will also need plenty of information from you. This will help her work out what type of care or support you will need to have a healthy pregnancy. Don't worry if you don't know all the answers to her questions. Many women do not know the date of their last period or about their partner's medical history. If you are not sure or do not know the answer, just say so. The most important thing is to try and be as accurate as you can, especially about things such as smoking or taking drugs. All information is confidential and is only used to make sure that the right care is provided for you and your baby.

GENERAL TIPS

Always make an appointment to see your GP, midwife or practice nurse.

Avoid making non-urgent appointments on Monday mornings or after bank holidays.

Tell the receptionist you wish to see your own GP.

Make a list of any issues you want to discuss. Put the one that is worrying you at the top.

Take your partner, friend or relative along if you want some support.

Be ready to ask questions.

Wear clothing that is manageable if you need to be examined or weighed.

Cancel appointments if you cannot attend.

TELL YOUR MIDWIFE OR DOCTOR IF ...

You have had a miscarriage or problems in a previous pregnancy

You have a medical condition which means that you are taking drugs e.g. epilepsy, asthma, diabetes

You or your partner has a family history of a inherited disease such as cystic fibrosis

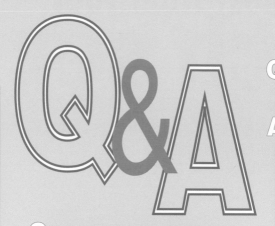

Q What should I do if I don't get on with my GP or midwife?

A Although rare, some women do want to change GP or midwife. This is quite straightforward to do and best done as early on in the pregnancy as possible. This means that the new person taking over your care will know more about you and your needs. To switch GP, you can ask to join the list of another GP in the practice or visit another surgery and ask to join the list. If you have any difficulties in doing this, you should write to the local Area Family Practitioner Committee. Their number can be found in the yellow pages. If you do not feel comfortable with the midwife that has been assigned to your care, you should talk to your doctor. In large GP practices, there are often a team of midwives working and so changing should not be a problem. In smaller practices, your GP should be able to arrange for you to visit another midwife.

Q The father of the baby is not my partner. Do I have to say anything?

A Everything that you say to a midwife or doctor is confidential. Doctors and midwives are able to do their jobs better when they are given information by patients. Ideally, you should say something because the baby will be carrying the father's genes and some medical conditions can be inherited. The choice as to whether or not you say something will however be completely down to you.

Q Do I have to have blood tests?

A While few people enjoy giving blood, it is essential that a sample is taken as part of your care. Blood that is taken is checked to find out your blood group and also whether your blood is rhesus negative. Pregnant women who are rhesus negative can have miscarriages in later pregnancies and so are treated with a simple injection. Your blood is also screened for some infections so that you can be treated or your baby can be immunised at birth. You may also be offered HIV screening as it is thought that as many as 10% of women may be positive without knowing it. It is possible to prevent a baby from becoming infected, so this test may be worth considering.

TIPS FOR ATTENDING YOUR ANTENATAL APPOINTMENTS

When you make an antenatal appointment, find out if a urine sample will be needed

Remember to take your card with you

Q I hate undressing and showing people my body. I don't know how I will cope.

A Firstly, it may be reassuring to know that no one can examine you without your consent. It is important that you allow your midwife or doctor to examine you because they will gain a lot of information about the development of your baby and your ability to give birth. This mostly involves feeling your abdomen (tummy) and can be done while you are partially dressed. Tell your midwife or doctor at your first appointment that you are worried about undressing. They should be understanding and this will make it easier for you. You could also take someone such as a friend or relative with you. In practical terms, choose clothing that allows you to undress partially such as a skirt and top rather than a dress.

On your first visit your midwife is likely to

- Ask the date of your last period
- Check your weight
- Carry out a urine test
- Take your blood pressure
- Take a blood sample so that routine tests can be done
- Ask about your family's medical history and that of your partner e.g. are there any twins in the family
- Ask if you smoke or take any medicines or drugs
- Find out about your work or other potential stresses
- Give you advice about how best you can care for yourself
- Provide you with an antenatal record card
- Arrange your next appointment
- Talk through any concerns that you may have
- Provide you with information about health services

Team list

Our quick guide to knowing who you might meet

PREGNANT WOMEN GET THE SUPPORT AND HELP OF A TEAM OF SPECIALISED PEOPLE. YOUR GP AND COMMUNITY MIDWIFE ARE THE KEY PLAYERS IN THIS TEAM AND WILL ORGANISE YOUR CARE.

Community midwife	Community midwives are often attached to GP surgeries. Your community midwife will get to know you during the pregnancy and also look after you in the early days after you have given birth at home. A midwife may also be present at the birth.
Dietician	Dieticians provide advice about food and nutrition. If you have diabetes or need some advice with diet, your midwife or doctor may offer you an appointment with them.
Doctor , GP (General Practitioner)	Family doctors are trained in most aspects of medicine. They can provide general and medical care, but will refer you to the community midwife or obstetrician for more specialised care.
Gynaecologist	Gynaecologists are doctors who have specialised in the health of women's reproductive organs. If you have difficulty in conceiving or for example heavy periods, your doctor may refer you to a gynaecologist. Many gynaecologists also specialise in obsetrics.
Health Visitor	Health visitors are trained nurses who have specialised in the health of the whole family. Health visitors are often attached to GPs surgeries or health clinics. Your health visitor will contact you either before or just after you have given birth. They will give you support and advice once your baby is born.
Hospital midwife	Hospital midwives deliver babies in hospitals, provide antenatal care and advice and also support women in hospital before and after they have given birth.
Obstetrician	Obstetricians are doctors who have specialised in the care of pregnant women. The most senior obstetricians in hospitals are called consultants. Most women see an obstetrician at some point in the pregnancy, although if a pregnancy and birth is without complications, care will be the responsibility of midwives. Many obstetricians also specialise in gynaecology.
Paediatrician	Paediatricians are doctors who have specialised in the care of babies and children. Most hospitals use paediatricians to routinely check newborn babies.
Physiotherapist	Physiotherapists are trained to assess, treat and also prevent difficulties in movement. If you have a pre-existing back problem or difficulty in moving, you may be referred to see a physiotherapist who will help you during the pregnancy. Physiotherapists are often involved in antenatal classes to give advice about coping with birth and also getting fit afterwards.
Radiographer	During your pregnancy, you will be offered at least one ultrasound scan. These are usually carried out by radiographers or specialist midwives and nurses.

Sources of information

Organisations in the following list may be able to answer specific questions you have that are not covered in this book. They are grouped into sections to help you easily find the organisation most appropriate to your request.

For further information from Tommy's, please contact:
Information Department
Tommy's, the baby charity
Nicholas House
3 Laurence Pountney Hill
London EC4R 0BB
Information line: 0870 777 30 60
Email: info@tommys.org   Website: www.tommys.org

General Support

Citizens Advice Bureau
www.nacab.org.uk
www.adviceguide.org.uk
Check local phone directory or the website for your nearest office.
Help people solve problems, including debt and consumer issues, benefits, housing, legal matters, employment, and immigration. Advisers can help fill out forms, write letters, negotiate with creditors and represent clients at court or tribunal. Information and advice available in a variety of languages.

NHS Direct
www.nhsdirect.nhs.uk
24 hour nurse-led helpline providing confidential healthcare advice and information
0845 46 47.

Relate
Herbert Gray College
Little Church Street
Rugby
Warwickshire CV21 3AP
Tel: 0845 130 40 10
www.relate.org.uk
Confidential counselling on relationship problems.

Samaritans
The Upper Mill
Kingston Road
Ewell
Surrey KT17 2AF
Tel: 08457 90 90 90
www.samaritans.org.uk
Confidential emotional support for anyone in crisis.

Women's Health Information Centre
52 Featherstone Street, London EC1Y 8RT
Tel: 020 7251 6333

Helpline 0845 125 5254
(Mon–Fri 9.30am–1.30pm)
www.womenshealthlondon.org.uk
Provides health information and advice on a wide range of women's health issues.

Alcohol, Drugs & Smoking

Alcoholics Anonymous
PO Box 1
Stonebow House
Stonebow
York YO1 7NJ
Tel: 0845 769 7555
www.alcoholics-anonymous.org.uk
Self-help groups where members encourage each other to stop drinking and to stay off drink. For your nearest group look in the phone book or contact the General Service Office.

Alcohol Concern
Waterbridge House
32–36 Loman Street
London SE1 0EE
Tel: 020 7922 8663
www.alcoholconcern.org.uk

Drinkline
www.wrecked.co.uk
Information and support line 0800 917 8282 (Thurs–Sat 24 hours, Sun–Wed 7am–11pm). Offers support and information about alcohol related concerns.

National Drugs Helpline
Tel: 0800 77 66 00
www.talktofrank.com
Advice and information is given by trained advisors on local services available and offers support for drug related problems.

NHS Pregnancy smoking helpline
Tel: 0800 169 9 169
Confidential helpline providing support, advice and information for pregnant women or those trying to get pregnant wanting to stop smoking

NHS Smoking helpline
Tel: 0800 169 0 169
www.givingupsmoking.co.uk

Family Planning

British Pregnancy Advisory Service
Austy Manor
Wootton Wawen
Solihull
West Midlands B95 6BX
Tel: 08457 30 40 30
www.bpas.org
Provides a confidential counselling and information service for women who are unsure whether to continue with a pregnancy.

Brook Advisory Centres
421 Highgate Studios
53–79 Highgate Road
London NW5 1TL
Helpline for contraceptive advice
0800 0185 023
Tel: 020 7284 6040
www.brook.org.uk
Brook Advisory Centres (commonly known just as Brook) provides free and confidential sexual health advice and services for young people (specifically aged under 25) and provides supplies via centres across the country.

fpa (Family Planning Association)
2–12 Pentonville Road
London N1 9FP
Helpline: 0845 310 1334
(Mon–Fri 9am–7pm)
Tel: 020 7837 5432
www.fpa.org.uk
Provides a confidential advice service on sexual health and reproductive issues for people throughout the UK.

Pre-pregnancy

Foresight
28 The Paddock
Godalming
Surrey GU7 1XD
Tel: 01483 427839
www.foresight-preconception.org.uk
Aims to promote the importance of good health and nutritional status in both parents before

conceiving a baby, and to provide sensible, acheivable information and advice on how to do this.

Infertility

CHILD – National Infertility Support Network
Charter House
43 St Leonards Road
Bexhill on Sea
East Sussex TN40 1JA
Tel: 01424 732361 (Mon–Fri 9am–5.30pm)
www.child.org.uk
Helpline for people with infertility-related problems. Offers advice, information, support and a listening ear, plus produces a range of factsheets on specific types of infertility.

ISSUE (The National Fertility Association)
114 Lichfield Street
Walsall
West Midlands WS1 1SZ
Tel: 01922 722888
www.issue.co.uk
24 hour helpline for people with fertility problems. Telephone counselling available (Mon–Thurs 7.30–9.30pm and Friday 8–10pm)

Verity – The Polycystic Ovaries Self-Help Group
52–54 Featherstone Street
London EC1Y 8RT
www.verity-pcos.org.uk
A self-help organisation for women whose lives are affected by Polycystic Ovary Syndrome (PCOS).

Parent Support

Gingerbread
7 Sovereign Close
Sovereign Court
London E1W 3HW
Tel: 0800 018 4318
www.gingerbread.org.uk
Self-help association for one parent families.

National Childbirth Trust
Alexandra House
Oldham Terrace
Acton
London W3 6NH
Enquiry line 0870 444 8707 (Mon–Fri 9am–5pm), Breastfeeding line 0870 444 8708 (every day 8am–10pm).
www.nct-online.org
Provides information and support to new parents during childbirth and early parenthood.

Complementary medicine

British Medical Acupuncture Society
12 Marbury House
Higher Whitley
Warrington
Cheshire WA4 4QW
Tel: 01925 730727
www.medical-acupuncture.co.uk

British Acupuncture Council
63 Jeddo Road
London W12 9HQ
Tel: 020 8735 0400
www.acupuncture.org.uk

British Society of Clinical Hypnosis
Tel: 01262 403103
fmp.bsch.org.uk

British Hypnotherapy Association
Tel: 020 7723 4443

Working & pregnancy

Acas (Advisory Conciliation and Arbitration Service)
ACAS Head Office
Brandon House
180 Borough High Street
London SE1 1LW
Acas helpline: 08457 474747
www.acas.org.uk
Provides advice for employees and employers on how to avoid disputes through good practice.

Department for Work and Pensions
Correspondence Unit
Room 540, The Adelphi
1–11 John Adam Street
London WC2N 6HT
www.dwp.gov.uk
020 7712 2171 (Mon–Fri 9.00am–5.00pm)
For employees claiming social security.

Department of Trade and Industry
DTI Enquiry Unit
1 Victoria Street
London SW1H 0ET
www.dti.gov.uk/workingparents
Guidance on laws for working parents, including maternity, paternity and parental leave and the right to request flexible working. Information and advice available in a number of languages.

Tiger (Tailored Interactive Guidance on Employment Rights)
www.tiger.gov.uk
Interactive guidance on employment rights including National Minimum wage, maternity or paternity rights, adoption rights or flexible working rights. Also includes an interactive calculator to help parents and employers work out leave and pay entitlements.

Equal Opportunities Commission (EOC)
Arndale House
Arndale Centre
Manchester M4 3EQ
Tel: 0845 601 5901 (free, confidential helpline)
www.eoc.org.uk
Gives advice to anyone who feels they have been unfairly treated because of their sex.

Health and Safety Executive
Caerphilly Business Park
Caerphilly
CF83 3GG
Tel: 08701 545500
www.hse.gov.uk/mothers
Provide detailed information, in the form of printed booklets, about how a risk assessment can be conducted and lists risks specific to pregnant employees according to their industry. Some booklets are available free from the HSE website, others are available for purchase.

Inland Revenue
Tel: 0845 609 5000
www.inlandrevenue.gov.uk
Check local phone directory for your nearest office.
Responsible for the efficient administration of direct taxes plus tax credits, child benefit, national insurance contributions and stamp duties together with the collection of student loans and National Minimum Wage enforcement.

Jobcentre Plus
Level 6, Caxton House
Tothill Street
London SW1H 9NA
www.jobcentreplus.gov.uk
Check local phone directory or job centre website for your local Benefits Agency/Jobcentre Plus. Provides a general guide to benefits you may be able to get from Jobcentre Plus and other offices. For more information contact your Jobcentre Plus office, Jobcentre or Social Security office.

Maternity Alliance
3rd Floor West
2–6 Northburgh Street
London EC1V 0AY
Information line: 020 7490 7638
www.maternityalliance.org.uk
Expert information and specialist legal advice on aspects of maternity benefits and rights. Detailed extensive factsheets available on rights for pregnant women.

Tax Credits helpline
Tel: 0845 300 3900
For information on tax credits such as Working Tax Credit and Children's Tax Credit.

Parents at Work
45 Beech Street
London EC2Y 8AD
Tel: 020 7628 3565
www.parentsatwork.org.uk
Advice on flexible working arrangements. Provide publications including an employee's guide to flexible working and free fact sheets.

Loss & Bereavement

Child Bereavement Trust
Aston House
West Wycombe
High Wycombe
Bucks HP14 3AG
Tel: 01494 446648
www.childbereavement.org.uk
Provides support and counselling for grieving families.

Child Death Helpline
The Bereavement Services Department
Great Ormond Street Hospital
Great Ormond Street
London WC1N 3JH
Tel: 0860 282986 (freephone)
(open evenings 7pm–10pm; Mon, Wed, Fri 10am–1pm)
Helpline for anyone affected by the death of a child of any age, offering befriending, advice, information, counselling, listening and referrals (also based at the Alder Centre, Alder Hey Hospital Liverpool).

Confidential Enquiry Into Maternal And Child Health (CEMACH)
Chiltern Court
188 Baker Street
London NW1 5SD
Tel: 020 7486 1191
www.cemach.org.uk
The Confidential Enquiry into Maternal and Child Health (CEMACH) was launched in April 2003. CEMACH aims to improve future care of the mother, babies and children.

FSID (Foundation for the Study of Infant Death)
Artillery House
11–19 Artillery Row
London SW1P 2RT
Tel: 020 7233 2090
www.sids.org.uk
Helpline for people with concerns about cot death, families bereaved by cot death and professionals, plus provides information on infant care and listening support.

Miscarriage Association
c/o Clayton Hospital
Northgate
Wakefield WF1 3JS
Helpline 01924 200799
Scottish Helpline 0131 334 8883
www.miscarriageassociation.org.uk
Provides information and support for people affected by pregnancy loss. Acts as a contact point for volunteer support workers and self-help groups throughout the UK.

SCIM (Scottish Care & Information on Miscarriage)
41 Merryland Street
Glasgow G51 2QG
Telephone 0141 445 3727
www.connectedscotland.org.uk/scimnet
Offers face-to-face and telephone counselling with trained counsellors, as well as "Telephone Support Network", (network of people who have experienced pregnancy loss.) Provides guidance and information on miscarriage and related issues.

Stillbirth & Neonatal Death Society (SANDS)
28 Portland Place
London W1N 4DE
Tel: 020 7436 5881 (Mon–Fri 9.30am–3.30pm)
www.uk-sands.org
Telephone helpline and a UK wide network of local self-help groups for bereaved parents and families affected by the death of a baby at or soon after birth. Provides information and publications for bereaved parents and healthcare professionals.

The Compassionate Friends (TCF)
53 North Street
Bristol BS3 1EN
Tel: 0117 953 9639 (open from 9.30am–10.30pm)
www.tcf.org.uk
Helpline run by and for bereaved parents who have lost a child of any age and from any circumstances. Offers support and listening, 365 days a year. Also support for siblings, grandparents, parents of murdered children.

Wellbeing
27 Sussex Place
Regent's Park
London NW1 4SP
www.wellbeing.org.uk
Tel: 020 7772 6400
National charity funding research into women's health.

Specific pregnancy conditions

Action on Pre-eclampsia (APEC)
84–88 Pinner Road
Harrow
Middlesex HA1 4HZ
Helpline: 020 8427 4217 (weekdays 10am–1pm)
www.apec.org.uk
Offers information and support for women at risk of or affected by pre-eclampsia.

Antenatal Results & Choices
73 Charlotte Street
London W1T 4PN
Helpline 020 7631 0285 (Mon–Fri 10am–1pm and 2pm–6pm).
www.arc-uk.org
Offers support for parents throughout the antenatal testing process and when a serious abnormality is diagnosed.

Ectopic Pregnancy Trust
c/o Maternity Unit
Hillingdon Hospital
Pield Heath Road
Uxbridge
Middlesex UB8 3NN
National helpline 01895 238 025
www.ectopic.org.uk
Provides support and information for women and their families whose lives have been affected by an ectopic pregnancy.

GBSS (Group B Strep support)
PO Box 203
Haywards Heath
West Sussex RH16 1GF
Tel: 01444 416176 (manned intermittently/answerphone)
www.gbss.org.uk
Offers information and support to pregnant women and families affected by GBS.

Hughes Syndrome Foundation
The Rayne Institute
St Thomas' Hospital
London SE1 7EH
Tel: 020 7960 5561
www.hughes-syndrome.org
Provides information on Hughes Syndrome (Antiphospholipid Syndrome or 'sticky blood').

Hyperemesis Gravidarum Awareness Group (Blooming Awful)
29 Windermere Avenue
Basingstoke
Hampshire RG22 5JH
Tel: 07050 655 094 (if no email access)
Email: support@hyperemesis.org.uk (preferable)
www.hyperemesis.org.uk
Support group run by volunteers, for women who have suffered from hyperemesis gravidarum (severe sickness and nausea lasting throughout entire pregnancy) in one or more pregnancies.

Molar pregnancy support group
Support Group Co-ordinator – Barbara Robinson 01925 262093
Currently offers verbal support from ex-patients and relatives to new patients and their relatives.

Obstetric Cholestasis Trust
Support and information line 0121 353 0699
Offers information for women who have suffered from obstetric cholestasis or who suspect that they might have the condition.

WellBeing/Sainsbury's 'Eating for Pregnancy' helpline
Tel: 0114 242 4084 (Mon–Fri 8am–4pm).
Offers advice on nutrition for women planning a pregnancy, who are currently pregnant and who are breastfeeding, and for media and health professionals

Index